I0156865

The Stobart Nurses

The Stobart Nurses

Accounts of British Volunteer Nurses During the
First World War

My Diary in Serbia
April 1, 1915—Nov. 1, 1915

Monica M. Stanley

The Retreat from Serbia through
Montenegro and Albania
Olive M. Aldridge

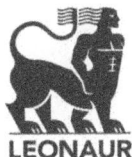

LEONAUR

The Stobart Nurses
Accounts of British Volunteer Nurses During the First World War

My Diary in Serbia April 1, 1915—Nov. 1, 1915
by Monica M. Stanley
and
The Retreat from Serbia through Montenegro and Albania
by Olive M. Aldridge

First published under the titles
My Diary in Serbia April 1, 1915—Nov. 1, 1915
and
The Retreat from Serbia through Montenegro and Albania

FIRST EDITION

Leonaur is an imprint
of Oakpast Ltd

Copyright in this form © 2014 Oakpast Ltd

ISBN: 978-1-78282-345-2 (hardcover)
ISBN: 978-1-78282-346-9 (softcover)

http://www.leonaur.com

Publisher's Notes

The views expressed in this book are not necessarily
those of the publisher.

Contents

My Diary in Serbia
April 1, 1915—Nov. 1, 1915

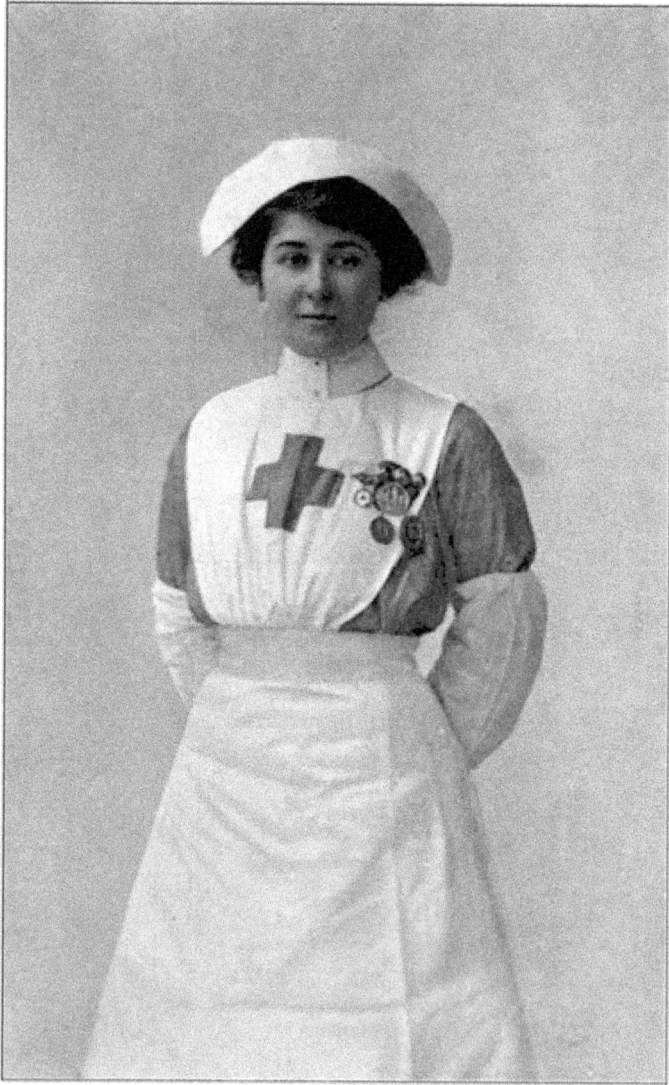

THE AUTHOR—MONICA M. STANLEY

Contents

To
My very dear Aunt
Elizabeth Stanley
this book is
Dedicated

Preface

Brave Serbia has not been forgotten in her hour of need by the women of England. For the Women's Imperial Service League, with Mrs. St. Clair Stobart as directress, went out to Serbia under the *ægis* of the Serbian Relief Fund, after arduous work out in Antwerp and after at Cherbourg. Mrs. Stobart decided that ours should be a Field Hospital owing to typhus and other fever raging in the country.

We left on April 1, 1915, on the Admiralty transport *Saidieh* for Salonica. The staff consisted of Mrs. St. Clair Stobart as directress, Mr. J.H. Greenhalgh as treasurer, a secretary, seven women doctors, eighteen trained nurses, four trained cooks, one dispenser, one sanitary inspector, an English chaplain and fourteen orderlies, of which some were chauffeurs.

The Field Hospital was perfectly equipped; everything we took with us. We had over sixty tents, 300 beds, with every necessary for them; bales of clothes for wounded and the civil population; the kitchen requisites, with four excellent cooking stoves with ovens; several portable boilers for hot water; large tanks for cold water; laundry equipments; medical stores; over £300 of food-stuffs; X-ray; all sanitary necessaries; motor ambulances. Our Field Hospital was to be at Kragujevatz; the tents were soon pitched and well arranged.

We had the following tents: one for X-ray, operating theatre; one to receive the patients; a large mess tent for patients and one for staff; one for linen—laundry; two kitchens—one for patients and one for staff; dispensary; food stores; a recreation tent for the staff, and one for the doctors; then there were lavatory and bath tents; the rest were wards and for the staff to sleep in. Our hospital was soon full. I was the head of the kitchen departments, and I looked after the catering and food stores. I was very happy with my staff, in spite of the work being hard and the hours long, but we knew that we were doing good to our fellow-countrymen.

Mrs. Stobart and the doctors found that the civil population was suffering terribly owing to the war, as there was a scarcity of doctors and no proper hospitals to send them to; and as we were trying to stamp out all disease before fighting started again, it was decided that we should have some roadside dispensaries and a civil hospital for all the worst cases. Arrangements were made that Dr. May should return to England to raise funds for more equipments. We also wanted more doctors, nurses and cooks. It did not take long before everything was forthcoming. Seven dispensaries were started and excellent work was accomplished in quite a short time. Over one hundred people attended the dispensaries most days, and over eleven thousand of the poor suffering population were soon relieved from their pain and suffering.

Monica M. Stanley.

SERBIA'S GREAT NEED

Mrs. St. Clair Stobart with Mr. Greenhalgh, doctors, nurses, and orderlies, were to have left for Serbia on Saturday, March 27. On Friday the unit met at 39, St. James' Street to have their photos taken, then at 4.30 a service at St. Martin's-in-the-Field, conducted by the Rev. Percy Dearmer. We had two hymns, a nice address; a collection was taken of just over £12 for our unit. After the service we went to a farewell tea at Lady Cowdray's, 16, Carlton Terrace. Lady Muir Mackenzie and several others from the Women's Imperial Service League were there. Sir T. Lipton, who had just arrived home, told us of his experiences in Serbia, with all the horrors and hardships. Lady Cowdray presented the unit with a Thermos flask each, as a parting gift. Lady Muir Mackenzie gave each a Tommy's cooker, which I found most useful. We heard that the Admiralty had again put off our unit, and that half of us only could leave on the following Wednesday or Thursday. The following Monday we had orders from Mrs. Stobart that nineteen of us would leave on April 1 with her (the heads of the departments, with one or two other members). We also heard that Dr. and Mrs. Dearmer were going with us, the former as chaplain to visit the sick and wounded, and his wife as an orderly to our unit.

My Diary in Serbia

Thursday, April 1, 1915.

Nineteen of the unit left for Serbia. We met at Euston station at 9.30. The train left at 10.30 a.m. for Liverpool. We had crowds of friends to see us off. All the equipments for our Field Hospital had gone the previous Saturday by the *Torcello* from the East Indian Docks by the Admiralty transport. We are taking out sixty-three tents; the large ones hold fifteen to twenty patients. We have 300 beds and all other equipments to fit up a hospital, with over £300 worth of food-stuffs.

All the unit are in a dark grey uniform with large pockets, making it most useful, and nice hats to match.

We arrived in Liverpool at 2.30 p.m. on Thursday; then collected our luggage. We were each allowed to take one cabin trunk and a hold-all.

On reaching the docks we got on the boat *Saidieh* for Salonika. We left the docks at 10 o'clock, and lay in the harbour till Good Friday, starting at 8.30 p.m. We could not leave before, we heard, owing to messages sent to the captain. It was nice and calm Friday night, but I did not take off my clothes and could not sleep, thinking and wondering if any danger might come to us. The *Saidieh* is a horrid boat, not at all clean, and the sanitary arrangements are terrible. It is a Greek boat of about 3,000 tons; in the usual way it carries mails and cargo to and from Greece and Constantinople. The weather was good as far as St. George's Channel; we could see Ireland when in the Irish Sea; but it became rather misty, a sea fog came on, and the horn was continually sounded.

Saturday, April 3, 1915.

The weather continues to get stormy, the boat rolls terribly; most of the passengers are getting ill, so we get fewer and fewer to meals.

At midday the captain gave out that no passenger must take off any clothes at night, and that boat station would be held on the upper deck at 3 o'clock; this did not sound at all nice. At 3 o'clock we all went on deck and had tickets given us for the lifeboats in case of danger. Fourteen of us had tickets for No. 1 boat, two for No. 3 and three for No. 6. We were nearly all separated at first, but I managed to get our tickets changed. Mrs. Stobart was delighted, as of course it was nicer for all to be together. It seems we were in great danger till we passed the Scilly Isles. Saturday evening we were a very tiny party for dinner. There are about 150 passengers on board, all units going to different parts of Serbia. We have some of Dr. Berry's unit; Mr. Wynch's unit, called the British Farmers, owing to the farmers collecting the money for it.

I forgot to say that on Good Friday we had a short service conducted by Mr. Wynch; we had the hymn for those at sea. There is Dr. Bevis' unit, a Russian one, and the other units are the wounded Allies and Admiral Trowbridge's unit.

Saturday evening some of us played bridge, two doctors, a nurse and myself.

Sunday, Easter Day, April 4, 1915.

Nearly every passenger dreadfully ill; only about ten people for breakfast. The boat rolls most dreadfully. We could have no service. A terrible Easter Sunday. I shall never forget it. I was kept busy all the day. In the afternoon the only one of our unit left was overcome with sleep, so she had to rest. The captain said that if anyone was not ill, they could consider themselves good sailors. I am more than pleased that I have not been ill. We are having a very bad crossing; every minute I think our end is coming. I have never been in such a horrid boat. We have no stewardesses, only stewards, and they are Africans—all black. The captain is English, and the first and second mates Greeks.

The other thirty of our unit left today; they go from Folkestone to Boulogne and thence by train to Marseilles, where they catch another boat for Salonica. Owing to our leaving a day later they may arrive at Salonica before we do.

Monday, April 5, 1915.

We are still having a terrible tossing. I have given up my berth and am sleeping on deck. The noises at night are something terrible, all kinds of things falling and smashing. On Saturday night I jumped up at 2.30; I thought our end had come. I went round to see what had

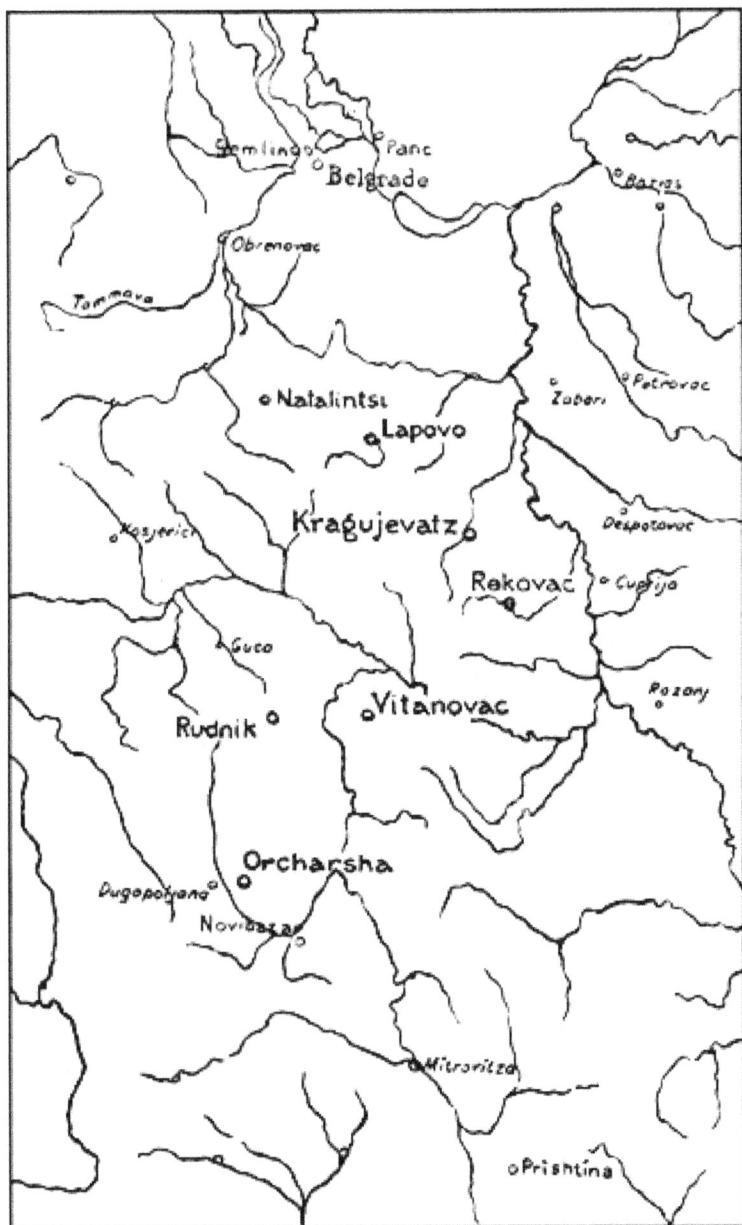

MAP SHOWING POSITION OF MRS. STOBART'S FIELD DISPENSARIES.

happened; the luggage was pitched all over the place. I have slept in the dining saloon the last two nights. The captain told us today that we could undress at night, we were out of danger of submarines, but I shall not until we are out of the Bay of Biscay. Most of us have been on deck today. I am hoping by tomorrow they will all be well again. Tonight about 12 o'clock we hope to be at Cape Finisterre. I shall be thankful, for I have not slept since I left home; the noise on this boat has been so terrific.

We passed Villan's lighthouse at 10 p.m. It was a lovely night and the water lit up with phosphorus. The captain appeared at dinner this evening, so things are getting better for us.

Tuesday, April 6, 1915.

All the sick are sitting on deck today, so we have not much to do. This morning I played deck quoits with several of the passengers. I learnt a little Serbian. We are a happy party; every one is so friendly. We have sheep, ducks and fowls on board—all have been sick; also two dogs. I slept on deck last night, a perfectly lovely night.

Wednesday, April 7, 1915.

The weather has quite changed; it is perfectly glorious today. This morning we learnt Serbian for a little and wrote letters. This afternoon I have been sitting in a lifeboat, with the sun streaming on me; it was heavenly. We have just passed Portugal. I took several photos. We passed Cape St. Vincent at 2.30 p.m. We could never have been saved if anything had gone wrong with this boat; it is a terrible old tub. We get to Gibraltar to-morrow, I hear, about 10 o'clock, so this will be posted.

We have just been having Swedish drill on deck, as the doctors wish to keep us in good health for the hard work we expect later.

Thursday, April 8, 1915.

Slept on deck last night, but always have to be up at 6 o'clock for deck to be cleaned. A glorious morning. Up at six, went down and dressed, then came on deck; it was a little misty. We could see Tangier quite well and all along the coast of Africa. Later on in the morning, and on the opposite side was Gibraltar. It was quite interesting. We were inspected, and the captain got our letters taken back for us. I took a great many photographs. We saw shoals of porpoises, which followed the boat for some distance. I took a snapshot of them. The day got hotter and hotter, so we sat in the lifeboat and enjoyed the view. We had to get out our shady hats, and we had no coats on. At 12 o'clock we had drill. This afternoon I have been playing bridge with the doctors, a perfect day. At 4.30 we passed the most gorgeous snow-capped mountains, Sierra Nevada. This evening the captain is having dinner with us, and after we are to have a dance. It is getting very rough again this evening, and all the portholes have had to be closed.

Friday, April 9, 1915.

A nice morning. We had drill on deck, then had our Serbian lesson. After lunch it began to get rough, and a great many of the passengers are ill again. We passed Algiers today, and we have a very bad swell on tonight, owing to being near the Gulf of Lyons. We have been playing bridge this afternoon. We had a dance last evening. Tonight we were to have had games, but it has been too rough. We have to learn two pages of Serbian every day; it is very dry.

Saturday, April 10, 1915.

A dreadful night. We slept on deck, and at 1 o'clock it began to thunder, lightning and hail. We got simply drenched. We are having it quite as rough as in the Bay of Biscay.

It is blowing a gale today. We are to have a bridge party tonight. We had an amusing dinner; we had to hold on to everything. A dish of chicken was thrown all over the saloon, glasses, plates, knives, forks, oranges and apples. We could none of us sit in our places. Great trunks were thrown all over the passages. It will be a wonderful thing if we get to Salonika. It makes me feel happy to think that I have so many kind friends at home remembering us in their prayers. I wish the Admiralty could be sent out on this boat. The food is nearly all bad; we can scarcely eat anything, and I hear we are getting short of water. We are not allowed to stop until we get to Salonika.

Our bridge party went off well, but it was a bit slow. Mrs. Claude Askew got the first prize.

The African niggers are very amusing; they call us all Misses. They told us if we did go into the sea and drown we should get plenty of fresh air, as we are so fond of having our portholes open in our berths. They will come and tuck us up at night.

Sunday, April 11, 1915.

It still continues to be rough. We are to have our service this evening. We passed Tunis at 8 o'clock this morning. We had a very bad thunderstorm last night again; the lightning was very vivid. A good many of us had to sleep in the saloon.

I am learning Serbian with Mrs. Stobart; she has just heard my lesson and given me twenty more words to learn. It is a most uninteresting language.

Monday, April 12, 1915.

Had drill at 10 o'clock, then "follow my leader" all over the ship. At 10.30 we passed Sicily; we could see the olive groves. An Italian destroyer has been following us. We erected the English flag, so they soon left us. I am taking part in some *tableaux,* so we rehearsed this afternoon. Since I have been playing bridge. It is dreadfully rough again, and we have another bad thunderstorm. It will be the greatest wonder if we land at Salonika safely in this wretched boat. I thought that our end was near many times last night. I did not get a bit of sleep.

Tuesday, April 13, 1915.

It is still stormy and pouring with rain, not at all a nice crossing. We did not see Malta; we were too far away, but we were only about two miles from Sicily. We have been playing bridge nearly all day.

Wednesday, April 14, 1915.

A fine day and the wind has gone down. Four of our unit have been ill, owing to the bad food (two of them fainted and were in great pain), and several in the other units. We expect to get to Salonika on Thursday, midday. We have just passed Belopulo; we shall be passing Andros and Tinos. Tonight we are all to appear in fancy dress. I am going as a mattress, a pillow arranged on my head, pillows stuffed inside a mattress ticking, and my feet coming through at the bottom with bed-socks on. The time has altered; we are 1½ hours in advance of England. It is light at 4.30 in the morning, but dark soon after 6 o'clock. We had a swallow following our boat most of yesterday.

The fancy dress was a great success; it was really splendid, as none of us had many things with us, as we are all in uniform. Mr. Claude Askew was very amusing, introducing us as Mrs. Jarley's waxworks.

Thursday, April 15, 1915.

It was a rough and very cold night again. I slept in the lifeboat part of the night, but had to get on deck at 2 o'clock as it was so cold and rough. We get to Salonika about 1 o'clock. We have just passed Mount Olympus; it looks glorious with the sun on it and snow-capped. I heard the guns in the night—from Smyrna, I suppose. The engineer took me down to see the engines last night. It is a good thing for us that we have had a rough crossing. We should have been caught by submarines if we had not, owing to the cargo we are carrying; it is supposed to be coal.

We are only forty miles from Salonika; we expect to arrive at 1 o'clock. We telegraphed for rooms at the hotel from Gibraltar. We expect to stay in Salonika a week, as we have to wait for the stores. We are all such a happy party, and all the units on board have been so friendly.

A Greek boat told us that there had been a big battle at the Dardanelles yesterday, but the result was not known. We have no wireless on this boat. The sunrise was gorgeous this morning; it is much finer today. I shall post this directly I arrive at Salonika. It is dreadful not having any news from home. I cannot hear anything for a month. We shall not be able to send our permanent address for some time yet.

The most dangerous part of our journey was the forty-eight hours through the Irish Sea. It is interesting to know that the boat has gone 1,000,000 revolutions to Salonika from Liverpool, and a revolution is 25 feet. As we got into the harbour at Salonika there was a vessel called the *Athena*; it belongs to the Germans. We arrived at Salonika at 2 o'clock; we had to anchor outside. The doctor, the English Consul, and the head of the police came on board. Twenty-three little boats arrived to take us across; the men simply fought, and we had quite a difficulty. We found we could not get accommodation at the hotel sufficient for our unit, so the captain told us to sleep on board. We had our tea and dinner at the Hotel Olympus. The latter meal the captain of the *Saidieh* had with us. We returned to the boat at 10 o'clock.

Friday, April 16, 1915.

The *Torcello* arrived with all our equipments at the same time our boat arrived. Salonika is the most picturesque place; it is so hot, just like midsummer in England. The yachts sailing about in the harbour are lovely. There is a wreckage just near. It is April 7 there, and in England it is the 15th.

After breakfast we took a carriage and went to St. Demetrius, the Greek Church. It is perfectly gorgeous. Large marble pillars and granite supposed to be extinct. The arches are wonderful and all inlaid with mosaic. Then we saw sarcophagus or some of the remains dating back to 136. The pictures all round are gorgeous, very bright colours. Many people came to pray. One little family went into a corner where there was a picture of Adam and Eve in the Garden of Eden, the serpent was up a tree. They prayed at this picture, then kissed each figure; they crossed the altar, and kissed each figure in the other pictures. Then we went to the Church Sophia, another Greek one.

We saw many more people praying and kissing the figures in the pictures and crossing themselves. The Baptistery in St. Demetrius was wonderful; there was a wonderful shell-like font under a massive stone canopy. A little distance away there was a huge bell under an arch. We then went into another church which was being restored. On approaching we could smell nothing but disinfectant; we thought this strange. The interior of the church was beautifully arched. We had not been in the church long when we found that the floor was a mass of fleas and that all of us were covered. We went into a courtyard and caught hundreds; women and children helped. We were in a most uncomfortable condition. Most of the houses are full of them, and also other livestock. One can see the fleas jumping in the sand in the streets.

Some of the churches are full of Greek refugees from Asia Minor.

Saturday, April 17, 1915.

We went to see the French Hospital. An English nun took us over. We also went to see the soup kitchens, and at 12 o'clock one hundred of the refugees came with tickets for soup. We helped to serve it out to them; it was most interesting. All of them wanted more than their share. After we met the remainder of our unit, which had just arrived by the *Lotos*; they came overland to Marseilles, then by steamer. They had all had the most delightful time, stopping at most of the ports. We envied them after our ghastly journey. Dr. Dearmer and several others of the party and I went into the town, then to St. Nicholas, a church full of refugees—a sight I shall never forget; each family had been allotted a corner, and they just sit on a mat.

One family was busy at lunch; they had one large bowl of soup in the centre of the mat, and they all sat round; father, mother and three children each had a spoon, and they all ate out of the same bowl. This seems to be the custom in the poorer quarters in Greece and Serbia. There were several little babies only a day or two old done up like brown-paper parcels.

In the afternoon we went to see where Abdul Hamid was imprisoned. He was allowed eighteen wives. He abdicated. The Germans threatened to rescue him, so high walls were built all round so that aircraft could not get near. After eighteen months he was told he might leave the country, otherwise be shot, so he went to Asia Minor, and now the house is used for military purposes.

Sunday, April 18, 1915.

We had Communion Service, which Dr. Dearmer conducted at 8.30. Then went to Turkish town, which is most interesting. We then went to the Greek military prison. Then to the Turkish Church. Before entering the church we had to remove our shoes; the floor was covered with squares of carpet. In the afternoon we went to St. Demetrius and saw a christening—most interesting. The priest first covered the baby, which was naked, with oil—head, eyes, cheeks, ears, body, legs, feet, back; then the mother poured a handful of oil over the baby's head. Then the priest took the babe and put it into a font of oil and water which completely covered it; then the baby was again crossed with oil, using a brush this time and taking the oil out of a bottle; then the babe was put into a piece of flannel into the mother's arms. She held two candles, one in each hand, and the priest took incense, which he swung backwards and forwards, and then went twice round the font. Then he read and kissed the book, and the woman kissed it twice, and the ceremony was finished.

We then went to the Greek cemetery, and saw where all the soldiers were buried in the last war. The Turkish cemetery was near by. We saw another large barracks and the Greek Military Hospital.

Monday, April 19, 1915.

We were shopping all morning, getting ready for our departure for Kragujevatz tomorrow, Tuesday. We leave soon after 7 o'clock. This afternoon we went with Mrs. Stobart as far as the tram went, then we walked to the beach. We were a party of twenty-four; we all had tea and then paddled and came home. I have just finished packing for Serbia.

Tuesday, April 20, 1915.

Got up at 6 o'clock, went to Hotel Splendide for breakfast; then we all marched behind a funny old cart, which had our luggage, to the station. I had a tin of honey, fifty-six pounds, which I bought at Salonika; the tin cracked and it began to run out; a cork came out of a paraffin bottle, and this began to *run*; then the luggage kept taking flying leaps off the cart: we had to keep running after it, to put it back: the man went on, never stopping for any catastrophe. When we landed at the station we had the time of our life, such a scuffle and rush to get into the train. Only twelve of us left to-day, and the other thirty-six follow us on Thursday. All the unit saw us off. The train left at 9.15; it was to have left at 8.

The smell of formalin in the train was very strong, and all of us were covered with paraffin, so the two smells *together* were not very delightful! Besides this, some of us had carbon balls and camphor in our pockets.

It took us about half an hour to get out of Greece. The country all along is simply wonderful; the most glorious scenery, hills, rocks and valleys, with the most gorgeous colourings. All along we saw herons, storks and eagles, vultures, magpies and jackdaws. All these birds are most plentiful and very tame. All the carts are pulled by buffalo oxen and donkeys. Most of the sheep are black; also the pigs and goats.

The train first stopped at Topsin, then at Amatovar and then Kara-suli; these are all the Greek stations we passed. The first Serbian station we stopped at one and a half hours. It was at Ghevgheli. There were many Austrian prisoners and Serbian soldiers on the platform. The Serbians looked very tired, and their clothes were very shabby. They are very badly shod, only a kind of moccasin on their feet. A good many of the Serbians have khaki clothes, but it seems that they have been given by the English. On lots of the house-tops and chimney-tops the herons have built their nests; this was most interesting to see. A great many of the soldiers have lambs following them about like dogs. They are so pretty.

Eight lovely peacocks were on the platform, and they kept walking under the train; also one or two white guinea-fowls. We saw no end of tortoises all along the line, and we got one and brought it into the carriage, but we had to put it out again as we had no green stuff to feed it on. All the lakes and reservoirs are full of bull frogs; these make a tremendous noise just like a lot of ducks quacking. The trees in this part of the country are quite small ones, and there are no hedges; the blossom on the trees is perfectly lovely. We watched the butter being made from goat's milk, and very good it is. Most of the work in the fields is done by women and oxen, and the women look very pictur-esque in their different coloured garments. We had lovely flowers all the way, especially poppies. We kept passing swamps, full of different grasses.

The mountains are wonderful, covered with snow, and we hear that when some of the snow melts dead bodies are found underneath. We crossed over the bridges which were blown up three weeks ago by the Bulgarians; we came through a wonderful tunnel cut in the rocks, and we passed no end of churchyards, where the men are buried in the different battles—Turks, Serbians, and Bulgarians—it is really pitiful to see them. We are guarded by soldiers all along the lines and on the trains. We passed lots of rows of little crosses where all the women, children and men were buried after the Bulgarian raid a week ago. A rope was put round their necks and they were hung up on trees to die. All the soldiers come and salute us at each station and along the line. They all look so sad. Uskub we stopped at 7 o'clock, and we were met by Sir Ralph Paget. We had dinner at the station: soup floating with grease and omelet as tough as leather; the bread was almost black and very sour. The room was very dirty, and many men were sprinkling disinfectants about. This amused me very much. We slept in the train.

Thursday, April 22, 1915.

We got up before 6 o'clock; had breakfast. It is much colder, and we are very near snow-clad mountains. We got to Nish at 8 and had two hours to wait. We were met by the Serbian Minister and doctor, and taken in a funny little carriage to the Reserve Hospital, where we washed.

This was the hospital which contained 1,500 Serbian wounded when it fell into the hands of the Bulgarians. We then had breakfast— bread, raw bacon and eggs; not good; but we must be thankful for anything in these bad times. The beds in the wards are several planks of wood, with straw mattress and pillows—quite clean. The women are not a bad-looking race. The minister showed us a terrible photograph he had taken of women and children hanging from trees, where the Bulgarians had strung them up. Two units we left at Nish; one is coming in a few days to Kragujevatz, the other to Belgrade. We drove back to the station; impossible to walk; the mud is eight or ten inches deep.

We slept in the train, three in a compartment, and none of us got bitten. We first cleaned all the carriages out with paraffin. We passed through vineyards and maize-fields. The women do the ploughing with the oxen. There are hundreds of wounded Austrians everywhere to be seen. On arriving at Kragujevatz we were met by doctors and officers, and were taken out to dinner. Four carriages, two horses to each carriage, a most quaint turn-out. The horses seem to fly along, and the roads are in the most awful condition; it was all we could do to prevent ourselves being pitched out.

We first went to the sanitary department and were introduced round, and then we all washed our hands in disinfectants, and were taken on to the prince's palace; it is now turned into a dining club for officers. We had a big dinner, starting with very fine Russian *caviar*. The dinner lasted until 10 o'clock. We then returned to the station and stayed the night in the train. One vanload of luggage had not then arrived, and it was too late to pitch tents. The bullfrogs were singing all night. When a Serbian introduces his wife, he says, "Excuse me, but may I introduce my wife?" When a party is given, the wife never appears at table. They must think it strange that our women are treated so differently.

Friday, April 23, 1915.

Mrs. Stobart has been with some of the officers to find a site for the Hospital; it is right at the top of the hill, and before the war started it was a race-course, and it was also used for sports. We spent the afternoon putting up the tents. The custom in Serbia is, when a death occurs, they put out a black flag for six days or more, and it was sad to see two or three dozen flags all along the town. We have been hard at work all day putting away stores.

The officers are most kind; they invited us to dinner, but we were all too busy to go, so they sent us a lovely dinner to the tents—some fried fish, a stew of beef, and a small lamb roasted whole, and a salad. One of the government officials joined us.

Sunday, April 25, 1915.

We had a service at 8.30 a.m., which Dr. Dearmer conducted, and he conducted another service at 2.30 and 5.30. Several of the nurses and officers came from other hospitals. The weather is very hot, but the nights cold. We hear the owls, nightingales and cuckoo all night. Several of our staff are ill. I have delightful people to work with, and we are very comfortable. Four of us in a big tent. They call me the "Little Mother," but my general name is Cookie. The government officials all call me Miss Cookie.

We have now started getting up at 4.30, breakfast at 5. We have had to put on our summer clothes as it is very hot. I bought five lambs today, 15 *dinas* each. They eat the meat the same day it is killed. The small lambs and pigs are cooked whole. Forty wounded arrived today; they all had a bath with disinfectant in, and then put on clean clothes, their own baked and tied up and put away with their names on. Some of the wounded look very ill, but this place will soon do them good. It makes us very happy to see them improving.

Tuesday, April 27, 1915.

More wounded are to arrive today. We are to have surgical cases.

When the fighting starts our Field Hospital is to move on with the army. We get quite used to getting up early. We are up at 4.30 and to bed at 9 o'clock; it saves lights. I sleep outside the tent, and many of the others do likewise. It is perfectly lovely. I shall never want to sleep in again.

The sun is glorious, rising above the mountain-tops. We are getting quite used to the noises at night. We have the nightingales, one singing against the other; the owls calling out; big black crickets, which live in holes in the ground all over our camp and fields, making their funny noise. Then there are fireflies, which at first I thought were search-lights, as they were so very bright; cocks are crowing all round at the various farms; stray dogs, which seem almost wild, visit the camp at night and try to get into the kitchens to the stores, and occasionally they will start barking and howling; in ponds near are frogs croaking.

My staff are so nice, it makes work so much easier. I went into Kragujevatz today to do some shopping. None of us are allowed to go on account of typhus, but there is not much fear when one takes precautions. The shops are quite nice and the shoes and clothes quaint. Singer's sewing machines are seen everywhere; also Sunlight soap, Colman's mustard, Peak Frean's biscuits, Peter's milk chocolate. These things remind us of home. Rice, haricot beans and prunes are very plentiful, and they form some of the chief articles of diet.

Wednesday, April 28, 1915.

The wagons are drawn by oxen; they only do twenty miles a day. They are magnificent beasts and are well cared for. We have bought two of them and have called them Derry & Toms, as Derry & Toms gave us two or three of their carts to bring out here.

We have had six officers dining with us today. The heat is terrific. I can't imagine what it will be in June. The Serbian food is very funny, but good. For breakfast they have a kind of bread-pudding; they call it our "English" bread-pudding, but the Serbian name is "*Popiri*." You put bread cut into dice into boiling water, with salt and fat; they beat it all together and serve. They like it so much and do not care for anything else; for a change they have stewed prunes and bread. They drink tea or coffee and the ones on special diet have eggs.

Sunday, May 2, 1915.

We have so much work here we seldom know the day or the date. We have just had tent drill, as we may move on soon, then we shall have to pull down our tents ourselves. We have lost several of our

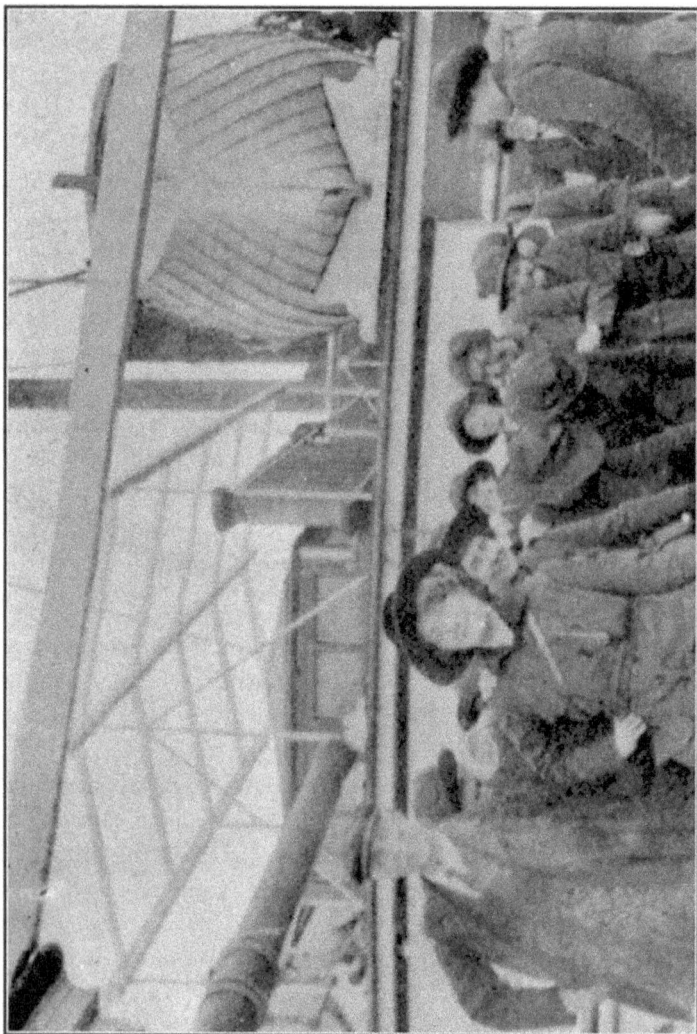

Mrs. Stobart and part of the unit going out to Serbia on the *Saidieh*, having Swedish drill.

stores coming out: all the bacon and lots of other things. Some of the men look dreadful and half starved; they seem to like our food. I have five Austrian prisoners working for me. It is difficult to get much work out of them, as they say, "No pay, no work"; but I said then there will be no food, and now they cannot do enough for us; they are not bad on the whole. I have a funny man who buys for me in the market. He is too fat to fight, and he is always telling me, with his arms in the air, that he works only for me.

We slept outside on our camp beds last night; it began to rain and the night nurses had to carry us in. It is lovely to see how the wounded enjoy this camp life; they are so happy. When they arrive they have a paraffin bath and their clothes baked. We brought a lot of clothes with us from England. Four officers came to see us this morning, and they lent us their horses for half an hour for us to ride. I am to go next time.

One of the doctors and I went for a lovely evening walk; the frogs were singing to each other, quite a different noise to what we heard before. This morning I took all my kitchen orderlies to have a bath, five of them.

Mrs. Stobart took our photos and I gave the men their new clothes. I managed to get them each a blanket and they were all very happy. They built themselves a hut to sleep in. They are all Austrian prisoners.

Monday, May 3, 1915.

A dispensary has been started on the road side near our Field Hospital, and people are coming for miles to get medicine and advice. There are many cases of diphtheria, typhoid, typhus, scarlet fever, consumption and other diseases. The civil population are suffering terribly on account of the war; they have been so neglected. One girl walked twenty miles to get medicine for her father, mother, sister and brother who were all down with typhus. A number of the patients come in ox carts and they travel all right; it is wonderful how quickly they have got to hear of the dispensary. Mrs. Stobart has decided to open many more.

Thursday, May 6, 1915.

This has been a great festival for the Serbians—St. George's Day— they keep it as a holiday. We had two of the officers to dinner, and a bonfire at 8 o'clock, and we all danced and sang; quite a good evening. The wounded quite enjoyed themselves.

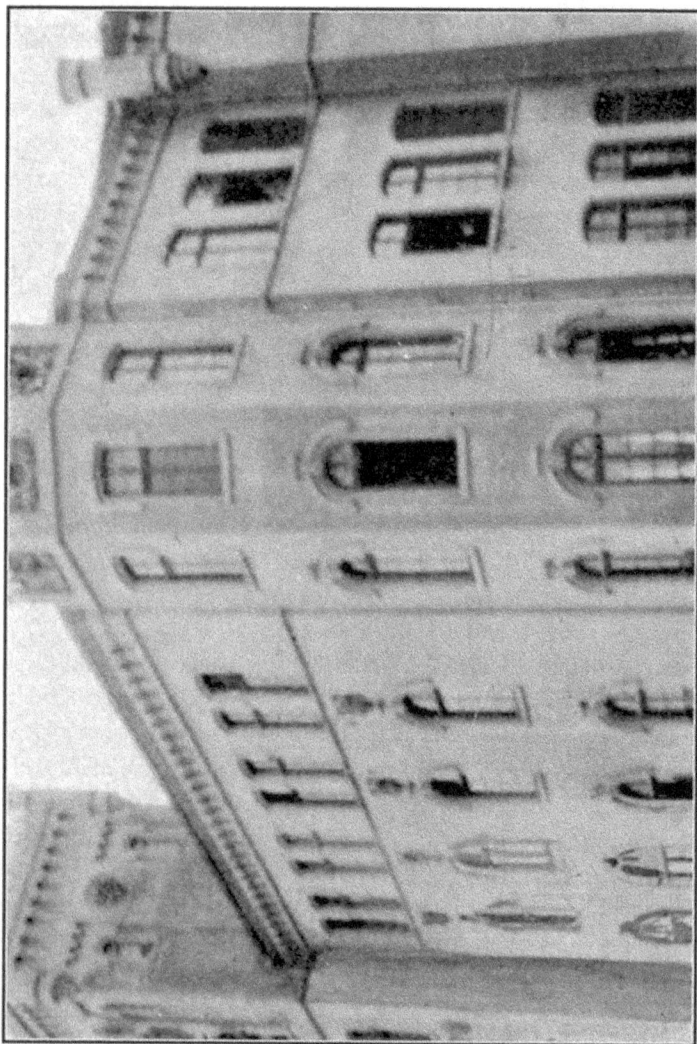

HOSPITAL AT NISH. WHEN CAPTURED BY THE BULGARIANS, CONTAINED 1,500 PATIENTS

Friday, May 7, 1915.

I went for a walk with two of the doctors to a cemetery near here. There are thousands of little wooden crosses where the Serbians fell in the last battle, also for those who died from typhus. The Austrian prisoners are digging rows and rows of new graves. The dead are not buried in coffins; there are several empty coffins lying about.

Many of the crosses have several numbers, so many are buried in the same grave, four and six. Our dispensaries are getting on splendidly; some of the patients walked forty miles; one can scarcely believe it. We feed all those that come a long distance. We had over 100 patients today. I bought in the market today ten sheep, six turkeys, five geese and nine ducks. We eat two and three lambs just for the staff at one meal; they are very small.

Sunday, May 9, 1915.

I was up just after 4 this morning. Mrs. Stobart and three Serbian officials went off to find another site for a dispensary. Colonel Harrison, our English military *attaché*, has been to dinner. I gave them boiled turkey and white sauce and macaroni. Turkeys are cheap; I got six for 57 *dinas*, and you get 36 *dinas* for a sovereign. After dinner Colonel Harrison gave us some very good records on his gramophone. Our gramophone has been lost.

The Austrians are still shelling Belgrade. One of my five Austrian orderlies gives me a lot of trouble. He goes off sometimes for three or four hours to get drink, so I had to report him; he has had his ears well boxed in front of me by the sergeant. If he had struck the sergeant back he would have been shot.

We have several wounded Austrians and one German. When the German is spoken to he always stands at attention; he is really a nice man!

The camp is quite a swamp. I got up at 4.30 and went to market with Mr. Greenhalgh. The market did not open till late, so we went into a *café* which was not at all nice; beetles were running about on the tables and floor. I sat with my feet tucked under me.

A lot of young wounded soldiers sat drinking whisky; it is only a penny for a little decanter out of which they drink. Other people had Russian coffee with a glass of cold water.

I am very troubled with dogs and cats; they get into the kitchen and steal the food. I have stopped the dogs getting in, but the cats I cannot keep out.

The wild flowers are very beautiful; we have different kinds gathered for the wards and for the tables; they are much finer than ours. I cannot get out much, I am so tired when off duty.

Monday, May 17, 1915.

One of my cooks has a revolver, and early this morning she was unloading it when it went off and hit me on the arm; fortunately it was not serious. The shot went through her box, then a thick pocket book, and thence into a tea caddy, where it remained. It was really very terrifying. A Russian and French military *attaché* came in this afternoon.

We have ten hospital tents and each one holds ten patients, and as they are all full more tents have to be put up. At 9 o'clock this evening a very bad case of typhus arrived in an ox cart—a poor soldier who was just on leave. His old mother and father came with him; they were to sleep under the cart, and as the ground was inches thick with mud, we got them bundles of straw; we also gave them hot coffee and bread. One sees some sad sights.

I went again to the market; it is very picturesque. Some of the gipsy women are very handsome and their costumes charming. Most of the materials for their dresses and aprons are homespun. The different shades of reds, blues, yellow and green are lovely, they all tone so well. We are just on 200 at the camp now, but the numbers never worry me. We bought cheese and great rolls of sausages in the market. My store tent is almost under water. I have had to put down bricks and planks and have a trench dug through the centre. We are told we shall have it wet for three weeks. The rain comes down in torrents, much heavier than in England.

The patients are all looking so much better and much fatter. I have bought two large copper boilers for soup; one cost 123 *dinas* and the other 77 *dinas*, but I should think they would last for ever. I have had a brick wall set round them and a flue at the back and a grate underneath. We only cook with wood; it is really very excellent as it retains the heat so long, and really I like it better than coal. But at first the smoke made us all cry until I got the stoves properly set.

Tuesday, May 18, 1915.

We have had an exciting day as the Prince Alexandra of Serbia was expected to see our Field Hospital. He and his suite arrived on horseback. The prince is the most delightful man, so very friendly and easy to get on with. Mrs. Stobart presented me. He was much interested in the kitchen departments, and shook hands with me three times. He seemed delighted and interested in all the hospitals. A Field Hospital seems quite a novelty out here. I talked to his horse, a charming creature called "Sugar."

Dr. May returns to London tomorrow to bring out new equipments, as we are to have six more dispensaries and a Civil Hospital. I have been doing out lists for new stores all morning.

I am having a lovely Serbian dress given me. I made some good Serbian cheese today; it is quite easy to make and it is really nice. I wish friends would send me newspapers; they would be very welcome. I picked up a cannon ball and horseshoe to add to my treasures. We had another bad storm; the rain drops are as large as a 2s. piece. It is really amusing when it gets windy as every one rushes to their tent to tighten their guy ropes, and when it has been raining some little time they have to be loosened. In the night it is not so pleasant turning out of a nice comfortable bed. But for all this camp life is very delightful.

The Serbians have been at war for the last four years. They fought first against Turkey, then against Bulgaria, and twice against Austria-Hungary.

Valievo was in the hands of the Austrians at the beginning of December, 1914. Then the Austrians captured Belgrade where they remained for thirteen days. On December 15 Belgrade was recaptured by the Serbians. Of the army of 300,000 who crossed the Save River, nearly half was put out of action. More than 41,500 prisoners were taken together with 133 guns, 71 maxims, 386 ammunition wagons, 3,350 transport wagons, and more than 3,250 horses and oxen. The dead and wounded Austro-Hungarians left on the battlefield exceeded 60,000.

Thursday, May 20, 1915.

The cannon ball that I told you about that I picked up was used 100 years ago against the Turks; there are no end lying about the fields.

Dr. May returned to England this evening; she will be away about six weeks. She will bring out more stores and will collect fresh funds for the upkeep of our hospital and dispensary.

Transport wagons are passing along the road near our camp all night, so perhaps we shall move on shortly. Oxen are used and they only travel about twenty English miles a day.

We have no fresh cases in hospital because there is no fighting at present. There are over one hundred patients at the road-side dispensary; each day some of the cases are terrible—typhus, scarlet fever, diphtheria, and a very bad case of small-pox, but there are no hospitals to send these sort of cases to. Today a poor girl arrived with one foot black, all the flesh eaten off her leg with gangrene; she had a tubercular foot which she had had a year and it had never been attended to. Women arrive with dreadful diseases, some with cancer.

People in dear old England cannot imagine the state of this part of the world; thousands and thousands are suffering and cannot get attention.

We are now trying to stop some of the dreadful diseases spreading, and are starting another hospital called the Civil, and this hospital will take in some of these bad cases. We are also hoping to have the six dispensaries along the line. Our Field Hospital is only for surgical cases.

Another wet day; we had a terrible thunderstorm which returned two nights running; the lightning is much more vivid than in England; in fact it lights up the hills all round and the sky seems to almost open.

Today is only May 9 with the Serbians; thirteen days difference; it seems so strange.

Today a man was seen buying Serbian whisky; he gave it to two of the patients and made them drunk. One of my orderlies did the same and was sent away last week. Owing to this one man the whole lot of Austrian orderlies were called into line, twenty-seven in all, and they were marched to the office tent, where Major Partridge talked to them all, boxed the man's ears who bought the whisky and sent him to prison for ten days.

There are three kinds of punishment for prisoners: first, boxing their ears; second, sending to prison for ten days on bread and water and solitary confinement; and third, to shoot them. It makes me quite ill to see the men have their ears boxed. The Serbians seem really good to their prisoners; I hope ours in Germany are being treated as well.

I had a lovely dish of wild strawberries brought me today as a present; the strawberries were strung on grasses and they are sold for 1*d*. a string. I also had a bunch of cherries and some sweets, and this evening two of the Austrian prisoners gave me their prison badges, so I was in luck's way.

All around our camp we have funny round holes. I discovered that black-looking beetles lived down them, but tonight I found they are crickets; they sing all night and are such dears. I dug one out of its hole and put it in the kitchen. We also found some of these funny holes where great large spiders live with hairy legs, and they spin such a nice strong web over their holes. I suppose this is their front door. We have been up to our knees in mud the last few days, and little streams run through our camp, but one gets used to these things; the ground is of hard clay and the water does not disperse quickly unless the sun comes out, then it dries up in quite a short time. This makes us think of our poor soldiers in the trenches.

Sunday, May 23, 1915.

This morning one of the doctors came for me to go and see an operation. It was a poor man who had recovered from typhus, then got frost-bitten toes, and they had fallen off; new skin had to be grafted over the stumps, and it was taken from the thigh. It will be interesting to see how it grows on the foot.

In the afternoon two of the doctors and I went for a long walk. We went about twelve miles right on the top of the highest hill, and from there, a few months back, one could see the battle raging from Belgrade. At the top of these hills we could see great holes where the shells had burst. Wild flowers are gorgeous. The acacia trees are wonderful, much finer than ours. Most of the hedges are acacias. The fields are covered with wild strawberries.

Mrs. Stobart and one of the doctors have gone to Nish till Wednesday morning.

The girl I told you of, who had the gangrene on her leg, had the leg off today. We put a little tent up for her; we could not let her go on suffering.

Another terrible day. I have never seen such rain; we are simply flooded; the storm lasted five or six hours.

Mrs. Stobart and the doctor arrived home at 6 o'clock this morning. We shall soon hear when our camp moves on. I cannot continue writing as we have another bad storm. The hailstones were like small marbles. We have now streams running through our camp.

This evening we had several of the officers to dinner, and Colonel Harrison's gramophone after.

We hear that the Italian military *attaché* arrived here today, and that fighting round about here will start in ten days. This morning it was interesting to see the transport wagons pass on their way to Belgrade.

This evening, while I was waiting for the last whistle to blow for lights out, I went a little walk to see the frogs in some ponds near by;

in one pond they were singing in a high key—I suppose they must have had soprano voices—and in another pond they were croaking as if they had bass voices, and as they made this quaint noise their jaws swelled out to a tremendous size. They came to the edge of the pond to see who I was and seemed to say, What are you doing here! The light from the hurricane lamp must have attracted them. The crickets are also singing everywhere; we can see their holes all over the hills. They work their wings together to make their quaint noise. And the cuckoo was also singing. With all these different noises it was quite an entertainment.

Friday, May 28, 1915.

Got up at 4.15 a.m. and went to market. I bought one sheep, some beef, five ducks, six kilos of sausages, 200 eggs, some carrots and peas. The sheep I gave 20 *dinas* for, and as 35 *dinas* go to the £1 it is not much. Ducks vary from 1-½ to 3 *dinas*. Eggs were 9 *dinas* a hundred and very good.

Wild strawberries and cherries are plentiful, but too expensive to buy at present. Market is over at 12. I got back by 9 o'clock. I have a man that looks after all the live stock we buy in the market, and he kills them as they are required for table.

There are three different markets—one for oxen, hay and wood; another for sheep, goats and pigs; and another for eggs, vegetables, cheese and fruits.

The pigs are all different colours, yellow, black, white, elephant colour. They are very tame, as they are made into pets and many of the little ones live in the houses.

On the way to the sheep market we saw a lot of guns, officers and transport going to Bosnia. The officers' horses had wreaths of roses round their necks; it is the usual custom, and the officers are presented with a bouquet.

There has been a scarcity of sugar in Kragujevatz for about two weeks; the other day they managed to get about 20,000 kilos, and at the shop it was being sold there was quite a raid. It was sold for 1*s.* 6*d.* per lb. There is no butter to be got; it cannot be made with the milk on account of typhus; the milk has to be boiled directly it comes in; it never tastes or smells nice. It costs 5*d.* per litre.

Mrs. Stobart has had a lovely bell given her by the Serbian Government. It has Mrs. Stobart's Hospital on it in English, and the Serbian crest. We only had a little goat's bell to ring to bring people to meals.

Today I had one of the Army Medical Corps Field Trenches dug, and it was most successful. We do not require it for cooking, but Mrs. Stobart wanted one made as they may be required at the dispensaries. I have already four lovely stoves with fine ovens and two large stewpans with wood fire under them. The pans are of copper. We have portable boilers for the hot water, which are most excellent; and Serbians have been to take the measurements of the boilers and stoves so that they can have some made like them.

Just been to help one of the doctors by holding a patient's arm while it was lanced for an abscess. I constantly regret that I was not trained to be a doctor. I am most interested in seeing operations, as one always has the satisfaction in knowing that the patients will soon be relieved from their sufferings.

Tuesday, June 1, 1915.

Sir Thomas Lipton arrived for 8 o'clock breakfast this morning. He had with him the *Daily Chronicle, Times,* and one or two other reporters. Two or three Serbian officers also came with him. Mrs. Stobart had been down to meet the train from Uskab at 5 a.m.

We had a very big party in the evening. Sir Thomas Lipton and many of the officers came to dinner, and afterwards a concert of forty musicians. The convalescent patients thoroughly enjoyed the evening.

We were all overjoyed after our guests had left to hear that our letters, which were a month overdue from England, had arrived.

I had nineteen letters, three papers and a book. I stayed up nearly all night reading them.

The sheep I bought the other day for 20 *dinas* is a great pet, just like a dog and follows us everywhere. We call it our mascot. It has a great blue ribbon bow round its neck which one of the nurses gave it.

Today our sergeant, who helps with secretarial work, has typhus. He has been sent to the Scottish Fever Hospital. He is such a nice man and has been with us ever since we arrived at the camp.

We had another terrible storm. I never saw such rain; if one is out you are soaked through in a minute.

Several of our members have high temperatures today; they have been isolated.

I have been to an operation this afternoon. It was to see a toe removed and two web fingers cut. I am really proud of our women surgeons. They are really excellent and so quick.

Friday, June 4, 1915.

We are still paddling about, up to our ankles. Two more members of our staff are in bed with high temperatures. We hope it is only malaria. Two of the Serbian Army Medical Corps came to see our camp.

Mrs. Stobart is still in bed with high temperature. I have to take all my staff's temperatures every morning and report to the doctors.

Two of Dr. Berry's unit have come to stay in this camp for a few days. Our six staff invalids are going on well, but they all ask for different kinds of food which is somewhat trying.

Lady Lethbridge is posting this for me.

We do not know what this fever is. Some of our staff and the doctors are beginning to think it is typhoid, but the temperature charts are most curious, not a bit like the ordinary typhoid.

I have felt unhappy today for our sanitary inspector has put disinfectants in all the ponds on the camp as the water was getting stagnant, and all the happy little frogs are suffering. Thirteen ducks from the farm near by have been to drink the poisoned water, and they have just run down to the kitchen gasping and their eyes nearly out of their heads. They have been given bowls of water and it seems as though they would never stop drinking. It has taken quite six hours for them to recover from the chloride of lime and water.

Sunday, June 6, 1915.

We had service at 5.30 a.m. in the mess tent. Two ducks walked in during the service. They made a great noise, and after the service we found that they had laid an egg just outside the tent. We had another service at 10 and another at 4 o'clock, but the ducks this time did not visit us.

My pet sheep had to be sent away, as it loved having its afternoon nap in the other tents. I did not mind it as I had disinfected it, and it was beautifully white and so clean; it was a great pet. I call it Sir Thomas. It was killed for dinner, and I went without meat for several days. It had grown so fat, and it was the best piece of meat we had in the camp. It was most painful doing the carving.

Tuesday, June 8, 1915.

We had five visitors today, four doctors and Lady Lethbridge. We again had turkey. This is quite a common dish in Serbia, and they are so cheap, only 7 *dinas* each; some are 5 *dinas*. Many of our units are down with fever; it makes us very busy.

Wednesday, June 9, 1915.

Today Dr. Dearmer and two of my kitchen staff and I went for a lovely motor ride as we have been too tired to go for walks, and Mr. Black took us in his car. We started at 2 o'clock and got back at 6. The weather is very hot, and in some of the tents the temperature is 110°.

Thursday, June 10, 1915.

At 3.30 this morning I was awakened by a gun being fired; I did not think anything of this, as one gets so used to the noise of guns. At 4.30 I dressed and went to inquire what the patients were going to have for breakfast, and when one of the nurses and I were standing talking we heard a great explosion. I knew at once that it was a bomb, as I had experienced the same thing in Antwerp. We then heard, as we thought, the Marconi working, and we looked above us and saw it was a German aeroplane. Then we saw another German aeroplane, and then two Austrian ones. We knew at once they were attacking Kragujevatz. They began dropping bombs first near the arsenal, which did not, fortunately, do any damage; then one near the King's Palace, which did no harm but battered several shops and made holes in the walls of the cathedral. The bomb fell in the middle of the road. Many windows were broken in the cathedral.

Another bomb fell in a cottage and killed a girl of fourteen who had only been in Kragujevatz three days; her parents had sent her from Belgrade as she was so afraid of the raids there. Sixteen people were injured and five killed. Then they came over our camp, a splendid target for them as the Marconi is only 150 yards away. The next bomb dropped was about 150 yards from our camp. The smoke was terrible; I felt sure some of us would be the next victims. Most of our unit turned out in their night attire. I was glad that I was presentable. The next bomb dropped was about 110 yards and the pieces were scattered all round the mess tent and the kitchen. One of the doctors came hurrying along and called for me to pick up some pieces of shrapnel, but as we got to the spot we found a poor woman had been struck. Her arm was quite a pulp; I do not think she will recover.

I got about fourteen pieces of shrapnel, a piece of the hanger-propeller and the fuse. Lots of trees were struck and I got a piece of shrapnel out of the bark. A wireless was sent from here and one of the aeroplanes was brought down.

There has never been a raid on Kragujevatz before. All the guards round our camp fired their rifles, but there were no aircraft guns fired.

We have not got large guns round us as there had never been a raid on Kragujevatz before.

Another poor woman was brought in wounded about 11 o'clock. She had a little baby which was *not* hurt; she was struck on the leg. The baby is exactly like a little old man, and it only weighs 6½ lbs. and is a year old; its bones are coming nearly out of its flesh.

Some of our staff who have fever are very ill, and some delirious. Mrs. Stobart is much better.

Dr. Dearmer is going to Salonika. He is meeting some fresh members for our unit, they are due on June 18. A Civil Hospital and some dispensaries are to be started. They will be branches of this one. The pontoon bridges and the regiments pass our camp every day. The weather is terribly hot.

We have started to use our mosquito nets. I had an arrow given me yesterday by a French aviator, one of the kind they throw out of the aeroplanes; and I have had a very nice Turkish dress given me.

Letters come from England very well now; they take about thirteen days.

Our convalescents sing and play at nights; some of them have very good voices. Their songs were generally battle songs, and relate to their friends who had fallen in the war. They are very clever in making their instruments—flutes, violins—which are excellent.

Just heard that some more aeroplanes have been seen but they have been stopped coming over here. The Serbian Government think that they tried to drop the bombs on our camp; we can be sighted miles away.

Friday, June 11, 1915.

Eleven of our staff are down with fever; it is getting quite serious. The strange part of it is the doctors cannot yet discover what the fever is.

We have 125 patients in the hospital, thirty-seven soldiers as orderlies, Austrians and Serbs, and fifty-nine of our own staff.

It was very funny the other day. Two large eagles were seen flying very high. They were taken for aeroplanes, and were immediately fired upon. The Serbians are quite ready for air raids, as we have some splendid aircraft guns placed in excellent positions.

Sunday, June 13, 1915.

The weather is very hot. I have never experienced anything like it, quite tropical. One of our doctors has been taken ill today; that makes twelve of our staff down with fever.

Mrs. Dearmer has been taken ill. Mrs. Stobart, a doctor and I had a conference about the disease. It was pronounced by the doctor to be typhoid. One doctor stated that it was due to flies; but this point was condemned, as the flies have only become plentiful the last week. It was suggested that it might be raw salad; but this was again knocked on the head, as no raw salad has been eaten for about three weeks, and then it was washed in distilled water and vinegar, and several of the fever patients never ate salad. The last suggestion was the camp itself. This is the most probable, as before we arrived this camp was covered with refugees from all parts; and with the very dry weather, and then the heavy rains, most of the doctors think it is due to this. Some of the cases have been pretty bad in spite of the inoculation. Temperatures are 104.8 and several are delirious. Fortunately none of the wounded have it.

We have had a terrible hurricane today, and a bad thunderstorm. Two tents were blown down. The hailstones were as big as large marbles.

Tuesday, June 15, 1915.

I was taken bad today with gastritis. Dr. Atkinson is attending me. I hope to be up in a few days. It is due to overstrain of the nerves. We have sent for five more nurses to come and help us. I have a lot to be thankful for that I have not got typhoid.

Wednesday, June 16, 1915.

Mrs. Stobart is about again.

Prince Alexis came to see our camp this evening. I feel a little better.

This has been a funny day, one that we shall never forget. At 6.30 a telephone message came up from the Government Office that we were going to have an aerial raid, and that we had better clear our camp. Twenty aeroplanes were expected, six were to throw bombs on Kragujevatz, and the others were going on to the Danube. All the patients had to be taken by one road and the staff by another, and they had to go about half a mile from the camp. Two oxen were put into one of Derry & Tom's carts, and patients who could not walk were put in, and these were the first to leave. Then the motors came round for the staff that could not walk.

Dr. May Atkinson did not want me to go; however, Mrs. Stobart insisted, and I was the last of the poor victims to be carted away. I was put on a stretcher and jolted down the road for half a mile with the other members of the unit, and we were plumped down on the roadside while others were fetched, and this went on until the camp was actually cleared. This was at 6.30 and the aeroplanes were expected at 8.

No aeroplanes came after all this excitement. Some kind member of the unit managed to get me some Bovril, as I was not allowed solid food. At about 10.30 breakfast was sent up, boiled eggs and some cheese. I expect this was thought a suitable diet for a patient suffering from a high temperature.

The army camp near was also cleared of its soldiers and oxen. At 11.30 a message came that we could return to our camp as the flight had been stopped, and that one of the aeroplanes had been brought down by the French and Italians.

I have five Austrian orderlies; their names are—Mike, Mick, Peet, Steve and Milko; they are really splendid, and so willing. They are all so sorry I am ill, and they all come round to see me and wanted to know if I was "too much sick." Mike works harder than ever, and says "Missis ill, Mike work hard, Mike good boy."

Friday, June 18, 1915.

I have been in bed all day but am feeling better. It is very hot again. Four nurses from the Farmer's unit at Belgrade arrived to help us; two from the Scotch Hospital came on Wednesday, and four have come from another unit, so we shall no longer be single-handed.

All the staff who have typhoid are getting on nicely.

Saturday, June 19, 1915.

I am allowed up for a little this afternoon, so tomorrow I hope to be about again.

Two great guns have been brought up near this camp. Two of the patients are about again. Dr. Atkinson will not let me go back to work again until my temperature has been normal for forty-eight hours. The work is very hard and there is no end to it. I hear we are to be sent for a few days' rest to another unit. We constantly have members of other units coming over for two or three days' rest here; it is so nice being friendly with all the other different units out here.

Dr. Dearmer has gone to Salonika to fetch the members of the new unit; they arrive tomorrow.

We have heard that the *Saidieh* has been torpedoed, and seven of the crew are lost. The Germans have been after this boat for a long time. We should have been torpedoed coming out if it had not been for the rough weather and the sea-fog on Easter Sunday.

The *Saidieh* had just returned to England under sealed orders by the Government. I am thankful that our nice captain was saved—John Reginald Ryall. We are anxious to hear about the chief officer and chief engineer.

I have a Serbian to take my place while I am away from work in the patients' kitchen; he is a splendid cook. He amuses us with his moustache; he keeps it pressed in a frame in the early morning. I think if it got burnt with his cooking it would be the death of him.

We started working this camp two months ago this Friday. We hear that Dr. May left England on the 18th with a fresh unit.

The baby belonging to the poor woman who was wounded by shrapnel died this morning; it is a blessing as the poor little thing had been so neglected. But the dear nurse that was looking after the baby was heartbroken. We called her Copper Nob, because she had such lovely red hair.

Most of the wounded soldiers have quite lost their nerve. When they hear that aeroplanes are coming they are quite panic-struck. We were to have had practice this morning with balloons; one man fled.

We have such a number of hooded crows here, and some birds called golden oriole.

Monday, June 21, 1915.
Nothing of interest has happened this evening. We still have crowds of visitors every day to see the camp.

Tuesday, June 22, 1915.
I am still not allowed out of my tent. I just feel like a naughty child who has been sent to her room. My temperature will not be obedient and go to its normal condition. Today three of our unit who have been ill have gone for a few days to Vrynatchka Banja to Dr. Berry's unit. When they return the doctors want me to go. We are just in the midst of another bad storm.

Wednesday, June 23, 1915.
Two of the second Farmer's unit have come to see our Field Hospital today; they are from Pojeropatz. We have the most ghastly thunderstorm every evening; the lightning scarcely ever ceases now; the thunder generally lasts about two hours; the rain comes down in pailfuls.

Thursday, June 24, 1915.

We have *The Times* Correspondent, a Mr. Robinson, staying here. It is interesting in the evening to see the little fireflies flying about all round the camps; they seem to be more and more each night.

Friday, June 25, 1915.

I am still in the doctor's hands, and am not allowed to work owing to my having a temperature. I have been in my tent nearly two weeks but am almost better. I am to be sent for four or five days' change to Dr. Berry's unit at Vrynatchka Banja. It is almost thirty miles from here, and a glorious place I hear. We shall motor over. No more of our patients have typhoid. Twenty-six of our unit have been ill all together; some have been very serious cases. I have had a greater power of resistance owing to my inoculation; most of those who have had typhoid were inoculated just before coming out here.

Saturday, June 26, 1915.

I have been allowed out today. Dr. Dearmer arrived from Salonika yesterday, with two cooks, five nurses and a chauffeur; he went to meet them from England. They are for the roadside dispensaries, so they are staying here for a little time to give us some help. Mrs. Dearmer has been very ill with typhoid.

Sunday, June 27, 1915.

Sir Ralph Paget has been over to see us today, also a Mr. Petrovitch. Five of the doctors and my two cooks came over to have tea with me. Tomorrow I am going away.

Monday, June 28, 1915.

Three of the doctors have been ill, so we did not get off to Dr. Berry's today. We had the most ghastly thunderstorm this evening, lasting two hours, such big hailstones. Dr. Payne, Nurse Berry and Nurse Newhall, Mr. Black and myself had breakfast at 6.15. We took plenty of refreshments with us and left the camp in the motor ambulance for Vrynatchka Banja. It is sixty miles from Kragujevatz. We came through the most gorgeous scenery, and it was so picturesque to see the women and the boys working in the maize fields. The women never wear hats, only coloured handkerchiefs over their heads, and if in mourning the handkerchiefs are black.

We had lunch when we got about halfway; then another bad storm came on and in a few minutes we could scarcely see in front of us for thick mist. We soon drove through it and came into quite dry ground again. The fields are perfectly wonderful with wild flowers, the most beautiful colours.

The hedges are all acacia trees, and the most lovely wild flowers. Butterflies and beetles are very plentiful. We had only one puncture, and changed the wheel and went on merrily again. We arrived at Vrynatchka Banja at about 2.30. We had a lovely welcome from the members of Dr. Berry's unit; six of them had come out on the *Saidieh* with us; several of them have been over to see us at our camp. We had tea at 4 o'clock and at 6 we went to a lecture given by Dr. Berry. In the evening we had some music. The other members of our unit which were here when we arrived left at 9 o'clock for Kragujevatz the following morning, leaving us three here for a rest. We saw them off; then Nurse Berry and I went to see the town, leaving Nurse Newhall in bed. This place is simply charming; it is far more beautiful than Kragujevatz, and is one of the fashionable watering places in Serbia. This hospital is very large and we have hot and cold water and electric light.

Dr. Berry has several other hospitals besides; they have only 130 patients. This afternoon I went into the large ward for some music with the wounded. We sang and played to them. The wounded are most grateful for all that is done. They call us all "*Sistra*" and often "*Dobra Sistra,*" which means good sister. The Serbian men look so fragile, with the exception of the higher class, who are mostly fine, strong-looking men. The women are splendid, so handsome and strong looking; they do most of the manual labour. The magnificent courage of the Serbian women will never be forgotten. Some have lost father, brothers, husbands and sons. These women have one simple answer: "*Sistra,* they died for their country!" Before such patriotism we can but kneel and pray for the simple faith which shall teach each one of us to be brave enough to do the same. Their country, beautiful and fertile like our own, is ravaged; disease, war and famine, yet they still go on. The Austrian prisoners do most of the work; they are such a nice race of men, and so willing, and never mind what they do. They hate warfare. We are all impressed with them. It seems hard that they have to fight against the Serbs. We went for a pretty walk after tea; we all went to bed early.

Thursday, July 1, 1915.

It is just three months today since we left home. This morning I went into the kitchen and learnt several Serbian dishes. My two companions were not well, so stayed in bed. I went to see them at 10.30 and found Nurse Berry very flushed. I took her temperature and found it 103°, and her pulse 116°, so I fetched the doctor and she has to stay in bed. I spent this afternoon with Nurse Berry, and this evening we were taken to see the town. We went over two hospitals, then through the park, and to the post to get stamps. The Post Office was closed, but the girl was outside, so she served us; she had not change and trusted us with 2 *dinas'* worth of stamps, which shows how the Serbs trust the English. The town is very picturesque, such lovely trees everywhere; the shops are very small. I bought some lovely coloured stockings.

A man in the hospital has to be operated on for glands and is not allowed food. When it was time for his operation he refused to be done; however, the doctors persuaded him. After the chloroform he was violently sick, and he brought up nothing but red matter. The doctors thought at first it was blood and they thought they had cut a vein. However, it appears the man had gone off and gorged himself with mulberries as he did not like being starved. White and red mulberry trees grow wild over here. I went to see a doctor at Dr. Banks' unit at the Red Cross Hospital for Dr. Dearmer; they told us the story that Dr. Dearmer had written in the English papers about the man who was thought to be dead and was put into his coffin. After the coffin was put into the mortuary the man managed to get out and was found by the nurse back in his bed.

Friday, July 2, 1915.

I have had a most interesting day; I spent part of the morning in the wards, helping with dressings. It is really terrible to see these poor men; most of them have lost their legs and feet; hundreds and hundreds of the men have lost their toes and feet through frost-bite; one poor fellow of only twenty-two has lost both his feet, and often calls me to show me the two stumps. It would be a blessing if some of these poor men had been killed right out, instead of all the suffering they go through. Most of them seem happy, and it is because they won't be able to go and fight again. Nurse Berry and Nurse Newhall have been in bed nearly all day; they are in my care.

After lunch I spent the afternoon in the kitchen, learning Serbian cooking; their method of pastry making is perfectly wonderful. They make the flour into a paste with water and fat. Then it is stretched over tables and it is pulled out until it is as thin as paper. This evening I was to have gone into the town, but we made a call on a French lady and a big storm came on and we did not get any further.

Saturday, July 3, 1915.

Dr. and Mrs. Berry went to Kragujevatz in the morning for a conference. We went into the town, did some shopping and had some raspberry drink and cakes at a *café*; we had a glorious walk back. This afternoon we heard that there was a funeral; then we heard a lot of wailing in the distance, so we put on our things and went to the cemetery. We met the procession of about twenty women with a lot of banners and baskets of food. It seems that the corpse they were mourning for had been dead some time, forty days, so it was just an anniversary.

When we arrived at the cemetery the women put the flags against a tree, then knelt down round the grave and began to wail and cry bitterly. Then they lighted candles and put them on the grave. They unpacked the baskets and put plates of food all over the grave—bread, rice, cucumber cut in slices, cherries, little bowls of jam, onions, little glasses of wine and decanters of water. We watched this ceremony for about half an hour. Some of the mourners ate the food and kept kissing the grave. There were no end of mourners at other graves doing the same thing. It was the most pathetic sight I have ever seen, so sad to see the poor things.

Sunday, July 4, 1915.

A very wet day; nothing but rain and thunder. After tea we went down for a sulphur bath. Such a quaint place; it was a round deep hole with running water only about six yards wide; the water was warm. After breakfast we went another walk up to the cemetery. All the food that had been left on the graves on Saturday had been eaten by the women who had been wailing round the graves, with the exception of a few apples and cherries that had been left on the ledges of some of the crosses. We had a lovely walk back through some woods. There are crowds of wild cherry trees laden with cherries, wild mulberries and walnuts. The vine trees are also plentiful and so well trained. The land is fairly well cultivated, considering that all the men are fighting. The women are splendid workers. This afternoon I went again to learn some Serbian dishes.

There is such a nice woman here as cook. As soon as she heard I was interested she said she would show me some of their dishes, and Dr. Berry's sister is so good in letting me go down into the kitchen to learn. We have been over most of the hospitals here; really very good, and they are so clean. The park is glorious, but it amused me to see spittoons all along the pathways.

Tuesday, July 6, 1915.

We went shopping this morning and came home through the park. After lunch we rested till 2.30, then went for a picnic as it was one of the nurses' birthdays. We did not go far, only to the top of the hill, but the view round was magnificent, the lights and shades so perfect. Just before we started for our picnic, Mrs. Berry, who had been spending the weekend at our camp, arrived back with one nurse to take me back to the camp. They came by train; Dr. Berry and another of our nurses came by car.

We heard some very sad news, and this was that one of the nurses was dead, Nurse Ferris, a strong healthy girl of twenty-five years of age. She was to be married in September. She was taken ill just about a week before me with typhoid. It does not say much for inoculation. Nurse Ferris was a good nurse; she had a bright cheerful manner and was always the same. She knew Serbian better than anyone in the camp, and could sing the Serbian anthem. It seems strange that she should have picked up Serbian in this manner and then be put to rest in the country. It seems she died on Sunday afternoon at 3 o'clock. She was taken to the mortuary in the town and then laid to rest on Monday. She had a large military funeral. All the staff from our camp went, all the government officials and the units from the other hospitals, and all the doctors from these parts who had come over to Kragujevatz for the doctors' conference. They had a band and she was buried near the other nurses who had died from the Scotch Hospital at Kragujevatz. She was only put into a temporary grave as, when the war is over, the government will erect a monument to all who have died.

Dr. Dearmer conducted the service. The last I saw of Nurse Ferris was the night before I came here. I went to have a peep at all our poor invalids. When the poor girl saw me she looked up and smiled and waved to me. I little thought it was the last time I should see her. Nurse Ferris and I always had little jokes together when she came to meals; she was beloved by all in her ward. It seems this is the first English service that has been conducted in a Greek cathedral; the prince gave his consent and sent his secretary.

Wednesday, July 7, 1915.

We leave this afternoon at 3 o'clock. This morning I went shop-

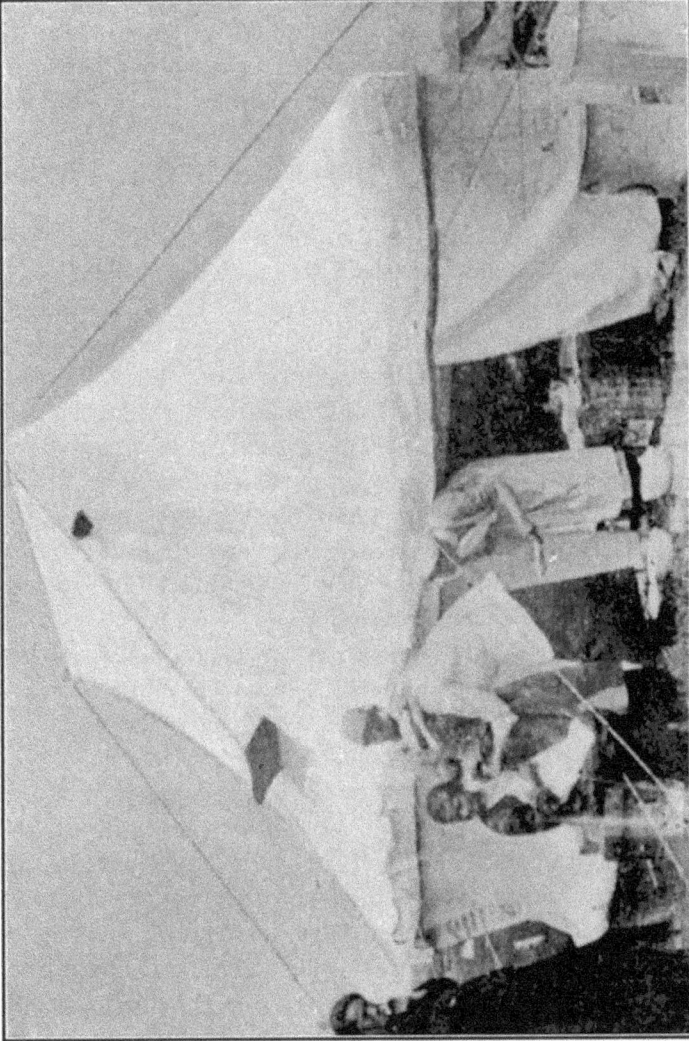

A CHILD HAVING AN ABSCESS REMOVED OUTSIDE THE OPERATING THEATRE.

ping, bought a lot of handkerchiefs and some Serbian pots. At 2.30 the carriage came to take the two nurses, who had come over to fetch me, and myself to the station. Nurse Newhall came with us, and Mrs. Berry's sister, Miss Dickinson. We had three miles' drive to the station; we arrived at 3.20 and the train was expected at 4.15 but it never arrived till 5.10. This is the usual thing in Serbia; we only have sixty miles to go. We arrived at 9; the train stopped at every station from 15 to 20 minutes, so the people get out of the train and sit by the side of the railways. It makes the journey quite enjoyable when one is not pressed for time. Our train was going on to Belgrade. We had two French people, and all the rest were Serbians in our carriage. The train was full of soldiers going to Belgrade.

The soldiers all travel in trucks, the officers in the ordinary way. I wonder how our Tommies would like this. We were to spend the night at a little cottage rented by Dr. Banks for the Red Cross at Stellatch. A boy at the station insisted on saying there was no such place; the railway officials wanted us to remain at the station, but we insisted on our little cottage and we soon found it in the dark. A very nice woman lived at this cottage, and her two children, a girl and a boy. We were put into this room with two stretchers. A nice Serbian who could talk French at the station said there were only two stretchers, so he sent up a third. We had a few sandwiches which we brought with us, then tucked ourselves up for the night on the stretchers, but it was impossible to sleep for fleas and mosquitoes.

We heard that the train for Kragujevatz left at 7 o'clock, so we got up soon after 5. It was very quaint on the way seeing little boys and girls driving along the roads flocks of sheep, pigs and chickens. All the children here seem quite grown up; the schools are all closed and they have to help in the fields with their mothers. The girls are very neat looking; they all part their hair at the side and have a neat plait at the back or wound round their head, and they have a handkerchief tied on their head. The middle-aged women part their hair in the middle and the hair always covers the ears. It is dreadfully hot.

On arriving at the station we were told that the train would not leave till 1.30. We have been trying to shade ourselves under a tree all day as it is too hot to walk. It is now 12.45 and our train is appearing in the station; our porter had just rushed up the hill to fetch us; it is not often one gets a train leaving fifty minutes before the time. We got to Kragujevatz at 7 o'clock, after a most tedious journey. It was so funny. Half an hour before getting to Kragujevatz I discovered

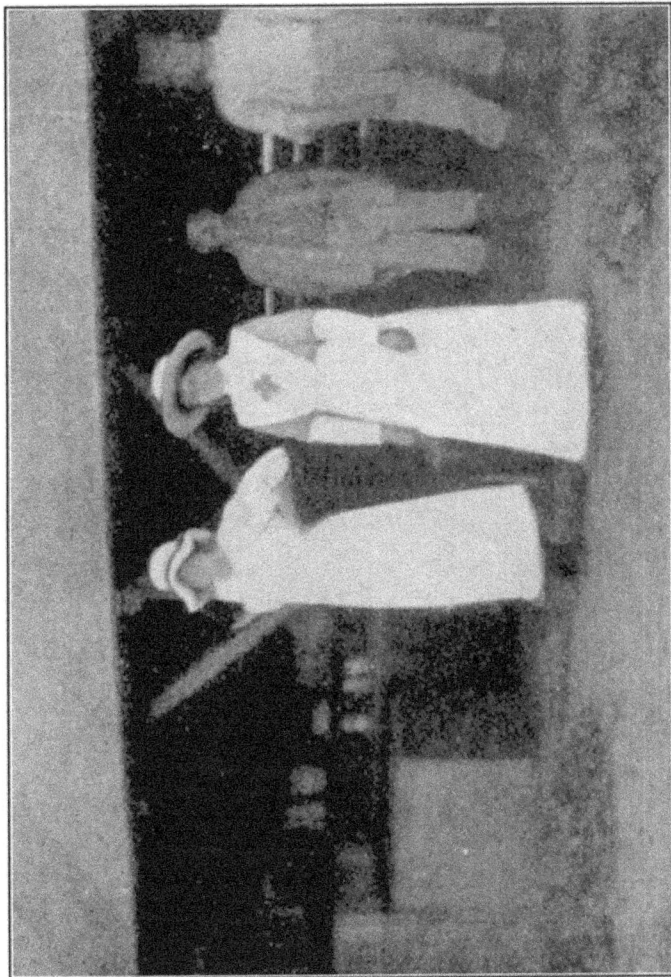

LADY COOK AND AUSTRIAN PRISONER ORDERLIES AT MRS. STOBART'S CAMP HOSPITAL, KRAGUJEVATZ.

that Miss Vera Holmes and Mrs. Haverfield were in the same train. It was so nice to see them; they were going to the Scotch Hospital, so they have asked me to go to tea with them tomorrow. On arriving at Kragujevatz we could not get a cab, so we had to telephone for one of the motors to fetch us.

Friday, July 9, 1915.

We had such a welcome back. One of the cooks is not well, so I had to do her work. I went to tea to the Scottish Women's Hospital[1] to meet Miss Vera Holmes and Mrs. Haverfield. I did not stay long as I had a lot to do, so many of our unit are ill. Mrs. Dearmer is seriously ill. This is the most anxious night; she has five doctors with her; she has typhoid and double pneumonia. Every twenty minutes she has oxygen given her; it would be terrible if anything happened to her; she is so nice and we are all so fond of her.

Saturday, July 10, 1915.

Mrs. Dearmer just a little easier today. The stores arrived today for the wayside dispensaries.

Sunday, July 11, 1915.

This has been a very sad day. Dear Mrs. Dearmer passed away at 7.30; she was buried this afternoon at 5 o'clock owing to the hot weather, and it being a general holiday it had to take place at once. At 7 o'clock four of Dr. Berry's unit from Vrynatchka Banja came to stay at our camp for two days. I have been looking after the invalid dishes for the typhoid fever patients. I made Mrs. Dearmer a large cross of some gorgeous white wild flowers with acacia and clematis. The Serbian Government sent up some lovely wreaths; the coffin was of silver and gilt, very handsome; it had the Union Jack over and was covered with wreaths. At 4.30 the remains were brought from her own tent to a tent we had turned into a little chapel; it really looked sweet.

At 5 o'clock the hearse arrived, a ghastly looking thing, with a statue of a man in armour seated on the top. It gave me a dreadful shock when I saw it; it reminded me of a circus; then all the government officials arrived, officers—the French, English and Serbian, and the prince sent a representative. Crowds of people arrived from other units. We had a military band; then the priests arrived, two in pale blue oriental satin robes decorated with gold, and one a peacock oriental

---

1. *Scottish Nurses in the First World War,* a double edition *With the Scottish Nurses in Roumania* by Yvonne Fitzroy and *A History of the Scottish Women's Hospitals (Concerning Service in the Balkans)* by Eva Shaw McLaren is also published by Leonaur.

satin edged with gold, one a rich velvet decorated with gold, one a red oriental satin edged with gold, and the sixth a black gown edged with silver. Each priest carried a candle, then two other men came carrying incense.

We all followed the hearse in twos as far as the Greek cathedral; all the streets were lined with people to the cathedral, and the cathedral was packed. The coffin was put near the altar and we all stood round. A large lighted candle was put facing the coffin and the six priests stood in front. They all took part in the service. I forgot to say one cross was in silver, with Mabel Dearmer written on it, and it had a large ribbon bow. The band played until we got to the cathedral, and when it stopped the people sang. The Serbs have lovely voices. They remind me of the Welsh. It was terribly sad; the singing in the cathedral was glorious; the service lasted about an hour and a half.

One of the French officers read a little address from the cathedral steps, then we walked on to the cemetery, about a mile; the band led, then the hearse and the mourners. Dr. Dearmer, Dr. Marsden and Dr. Atkinson met us at the cemetery gates; the priests continued their prayers in Serbian; then Rev. Mr. Little, who has come to join our unit, read our English service. The grave was lined with white and decorated with clematis. Mrs. Dearmer was buried next to Nurse Ferris. The coffin was lowered into a box, then the lid was put on. After the service Dr. Dearmer, Dr. Marsden, Dr. Atkinson went off in the motor for a few days. We all got into motors and carriages and returned to the camp.

Monday, July 12, 1915.

We have been busy all day packing and getting ready the roadside dispensary; this will be the chief *depôt*; the first dispensary will be twenty-five miles from here. The units for the dispensary go on Wednesday. I had the most lovely caterpillar given me today; it is three inches long, and is a most lovely green with lovely pale blue spots on it, and little tufts of hair come round the blue spots. What it is I do not know, and a man who is very well up in these kind of things could not tell me. I went to see two members of our unit off to Nish this evening. Today a Frenchman has been practising in a Serbian aeroplane over our camp; it is most exciting.

Dr. Dearmer has decided to return to England tomorrow.

Tuesday, July 13, 1915.

We finished getting ready the stores for the dispensary today. Dr.

Dearmer and Dr. Marsden left for Malta; Dr. Dearmer has his son there.

Wednesday, July 14, 1915.

This morning we were up at 4.15 as ten of the new unit were leaving to start the dispensary, twenty-five miles away; they left with all their equipments. Just as they were ready to start the Rev. Mr. Sewell arrived, and Mrs. Sewell from Belgrade. Dr. Hanson and Mr. and Mrs. Sewell and I had tea together in Dr. Atkinson's tent. This morning Major Potridge took me to the arsenal to choose a transport kitchen which the Serbians captured from the Austrians. I was taken all over the arsenal, which was most interesting. It is most wonderful the amount of guns which the Serbs have taken from the Austrians. Mr. Paulhan, the French aviator, is here. He won the *Daily Mail* prize; he flies over the camp very often going to Belgrade. Six of our unit go to Belgrade this evening for a few days. I hope to go before returning to England.

Friday, July 16, 1915.

Mrs. Stobart and three of the government officials went to choose a site for another dispensary. I was up at 3.30 and we had breakfast at 4.30. I went to the market to order things for the week. Sunday is the great day for the market. It is so picturesque to see all the Serbs in their quaint costumes. The gipsies are lovely. They have gorgeous striped skirts, homespun, lovely coloured belts with large buckles, home-made stockings wonderfully embroidered, fancy *zouave*, and fancy coloured scarves on their heads. One of the doctors and I were invited out to an engagement ceremony. It was really most interesting.

One of our interpreters who was single was told that there was a girl who would make him a suitable wife, so he went to see her early last week, liked her, so proposed. She is nineteen and he is about thirty-five years of age. The girl possesses a maize field, a wheat field and a walnut tree. This is considered a very good dowry. At 3.30 the interpreter called for us; the cottage where the girl and her people live is about ten minutes walk from the camp. On our way we met several of the man's relations.

On arriving at the house we were met by her relations, who were standing all along the pathway to the front door. The men shook hands with us and the women kissed our hands. We were taken into the front room, a good sized one with a table in the middle; there was tapestry all round the walls which had been done by the girl. The Serbs do the most beautiful work with the handlooms, and it is all done with the pure wool from the sheep, which one sees the women spinning as they walk along the streets. We sat round the table and talked till all the guests had arrived. The girl went round kissing all the women relations on the hands and face, the men and the guests on the hands, the *fiancé* did likewise; then the engaged couple stood in the centre of the room and had the ring presented, a gold ring with a diamond and ruby. The ring was put on the little finger of the right hand. The engaged couple kissed all the people again; we then started with refreshments. The girl did everything. A tray was handed round first with a dish of cakes and glasses of wine; this was to drink the health of the guests.

We only took a sip of wine and the glasses were put back on the tray; then the girl went out and brought in another tray, the same wine and cakes; this was to drink the bride's health; then a third lot was brought in to drink the bridegroom's health. Then a tray came in with two dishes of jam and glasses of cold water and spoons. We all eat a spoonful of jam and drank a little water; the last tray had little cups of Turkish coffee. After this we sat and talked; the ceremony was over. Fortunately we were not far from the camp as a blizzard came up with a terrible sand storm. We rushed round to help with the tents and patients. This was a difficult task.

We got our patients taken away in the motors to our new building near. The hospital ward tents stood well; as they are all double, only three came down, and the poles were not broken, so were soon put up. Fifteen came down in all, the staff mess tent, the men's mess tent, the kitchen tent and some of the sleeping tents. We had several of the military authorities helping us. The storm lasted for two hours and then all was quite calm again. We had a lovely picnic supper under a large shelter the government officials had put up for us.

The next day we were busy putting things straight after the storm. I was not well again, so was sent to bed. I had to get up in the afternoon to pack, as Dr. Atkinson had arranged for me to go to Belgrade to the British Fever Hospital. Four of our unit are returning to England, so they have come with us to Belgrade. Eight of us left for Belgrade by the 12 train. We had a through carriage, most comfortable. Dr. Curcin had arranged it for us. The English military *attaché*, Col. Harrison, came to see us off. A motor took us from the camp; we had a lovely journey and arrived at Belgrade at 10 a.m. It is sad to see how Belgrade is destroyed.

Our driver was too funny. The roads were terribly bad; we had quite a young boy to drive us. He jumped off the box part way to shake hands with some of his friends in a cart; he got a cigar from them, lighted it and then ran after his carriage again. We had gone on quite a long distance with our two horses. When we got a little further our driver jumped down again, this time for a drink of water on the roadside, and to buy a cake. We arrived at the British Fever Hospital at 11 o'clock; we were given a very nice ward, and the two nurses and I were sent to bed, and we had to go on light diet for forty-eight hours. I have been put on milk only, so I am very cross; it is very dull in bed, but I know many of the Farmers' unit as so many came out in the *Saidieh* with us.

Tuesday, July 20, 1915.

We have had a dull day in bed. Belgrade has been terribly shattered with bombs. This hospital faces the Danube; it is most interesting. The snipers have been firing a good deal today, and we hear the guns at night. It seems a shame that so many of these lovely buildings are in ruins.

Wednesday, July 21, 1915.

Still in bed on milk diet; it is dull work. This afternoon an Austrian aeroplane has been flying over us, and the Serbs have been firing at it.

Thursday, July 22, 1915.

At 3.40 this morning heavy firing started, and it continued for half an hour; soon after we heard aeroplanes; there were two Austrian ones which came over dropping bombs. They flew over this hospital many times. The Serbs started firing at them, and the shrapnel fell on the road below, quite a lot of it. If I had been all right I should have got some. The aeroplanes now have dropped a lot of sealed packets with long silvery ribbon which floated along for many miles in the air; it was quite nice to see them in the sun. We have just heard that the long silver ribbon contained a sealed packet addressed to the governor of Belgrade, saying that unless the Serbians surrender they will start bombarding the town.

It is the anniversary of the declaration of war on Serbia today. I have just had three more months' extension of leave from the Governors of the Institute, saying they have appreciated all the valuable work I have been doing, and have granted me another three months' leave, from the commencement of next session.

Friday, July 23, 1915.

Six of our unit arrived over from the camp to say goodbye to us; they were returning to England; they wanted to see Belgrade before returning. A few guns were fired at Semlin by the Serbs. It is splendid to see the way the Serbian women work. Some of the work-rooms at the arsenal were full of them, and even little boys and girls of fourteen and fifteen years of age. When the bullets and cartridges are finished they are tested in another machine, and if they have any defects they are shot out again. The Austrian kitchens are considered wonderful, they are so well fitted up.

Saturday, July 24, 1915.

I was awakened this morning at 5 o'clock by more guns being fired, but it only lasted a short time. Sir Ralph and Lady Paget called to see one of their nurses who is at this hospital with typhus (so they came in to see us). One of the doctors is here with an orderly to look after her. Lady Paget still looks very ill after her illness of typhus. I had a long talk with her; she is a charming woman, and Sir Ralph is very nice. There has been an interesting *fête* given today by the gipsies; they sent invitations to all the hospitals here. It was held in a large building. Several trays of refreshments were handed round; after that they played violins and some other funny instruments; they play and sing very well, but it is so weird. The French have sent round to the gipsy villages as their huts were condemned as not being fit to live in; but the funny part is that the gipsy quarter has had no cases of disease like other parts of Serbia.

It is pouring with rain and the streets are simply flooded several inches deep; the children take off their shoes and stockings and paddle, but most of the children do not wear shoes and stockings. This is the only place in Serbia where there are wood and asphalt roads, all the other roads are in a terribly cobbly state, and in a most deplorable condition. The shops are nearly all closed. Some of the people just open in the evening. The air raid we had the other day: a French aviator went up and there was a battle in the air; Monsieur Paulhan fired on the Austrian aeroplane and brought it down in Austrian territory; the aviator was killed; a photograph was taken after shooting.

This is the third Austrian aeroplane that has been brought down by the French aviator since he came here. We hear the guns each day; the French aeroplane goes over the Austrian territory, and then we hear the Austrians firing on it. We have some of our marines five miles from here with large guns, also French and Russian. The doctor allowed one of the nurses and me to go for an hour's drive today. We drove all round the town past the King's Palace. Some of the buildings are very fine but so many are in ruins. No trams or trains are allowed to run, otherwise the Austrians begin firing. If any of the nurses are seen near with their caps and aprons the Austrians begin at once firing; they think they must be Serbian officers.

Wednesday, July 28, 1915.

The French aeroplane has been flying round again today. One of the nurses and I went for another drive in a ramshackle carriage with two horses. When we got a little way the wheel came off; it was soon mended and we started off again, and the poor old carriage came to grief a second time, but fortunately we were near a blacksmith's place.

Thursday, July 29, 1915.

This has been a dull day. The doctor would not allow me to go out as my temperature is inclined to go up and I have a bad pulse. The Austrians are splendid men, and it seems so terrible to see these nice refined men doing all kinds of dirty work; it makes me think of our poor English prisoners in Germany.

I am much better today and the doctor allowed the nurse to take me across to the hotel where we had tea; it was such a nice change. Another of our unit came over from the camp to stay a few days. I had a letter from Dr. Atkinson telling me that Dr. May had arrived from England, and that Mrs. Stobart had gone to Lapovo to start another dispensary. Two Serbian regiments passed last evening, the best drilled Serbs we have seen since we arrived; there were eighty in each regiment; then a lot of horses and donkeys passed, laden with wood. I am proud to say that I have not seen any soldiers march better than our men in England since I left.

Sunday, August 1, 1915.

I have not been allowed out the last two days, as the doctor was not pleased with me. This is a lovely hospital, it will hold over 500 beds; it was an university before the war; the art rooms on the top floor are splendid.

Monday, August 2, 1915.

I have been allowed out for a little today. I went round to the hotel to tea with our nurses who were returning to England with eight of this unit.

In the morning our French aeroplane flew over to spy on the Austrians, so the Austrians fired on it. It was so curious to see clouds of grey and red smoke when the shells burst; it was quite different from the ordinary shot that had been fired at the aeroplanes before. A lot of the people here had a near shave of being blown up with the bombs. One fell just near a man I met yesterday and he was blown up four feet and not hurt at all.

Tuesday, August 3, 1915.

Today I had a walk round Belgrade to see the shops; some of them are very fine, but things are most expensive and the shop-people are very quaint, they do not care if they sell their goods or not. The sister who looks after me took me for a little walk this afternoon. We went down near the Save to look across at Semlin; we are not allowed to go too near, otherwise the snipers fire upon us. We saw the bridge that crosses the Save, which the Serbians blew up to prevent the Austrians crossing. We also went into several houses that have been ruined with bombs. We could see the cathedral at Semlin quite plainly. The sister and I went after to see the cathedral; the paintings are very fine. It is fortunate that—up to the present—it has not been damaged inside.

Malaria is starting here; we had four cases in yesterday. The doctor is afraid of our getting it, so we are to return to the camp tomorrow. I am not to go on duty for another two weeks. There has been much discussion in Serbia about our camp, and it seems that the site chosen was not a suitable one. First of all a camp should be on a slope, as I have always learnt from my V.A.D. lectures.

Secondly, the kind of soil should have been taken into consideration; I should have thought that a porous soil would have been best, but our camp is on clay. Thirdly, I think inquiries should have been made as to what the land had been used for before pitching our tents.

Another camp had been on our site before, and we heard that refugees had been living on the land for some time. When we arrived the land was covered with bullocks, sheep, goats, pigs, fowls, ducks, which, of course, produced flies, and as flies carry disease, I should think it was very unsuitable.

Friday, August 6, 1915.

I was taken bad in the night, so the doctor would not let me return to the camp with the other members of our unit. The nurses are giving us a tea-party, as they have had all kinds of lovely things sent from England. I had Sister Barnes looking after me, such a nice girl, who has travelled a great deal; a nurse who was at the Battersea A.V.S.H. for four years, also a doctor's wife, who is married to one of the doctors here; she is a Yorkshire girl, very charming. The three members in our unit return to the camp this evening at Vrynatchka Banja.

One of the patients produced an egg every morning for his breakfast; it was discovered that he had encouraged a hen to come into his bed, and then it took to laying its eggs. We have sixteen more patients brought in tonight with malaria; it seems to be spreading rapidly, so it is a good thing that our people have returned to Kragujevatz. All the doctors out here think that mistakes were made at the first when typhus broke out, by sending the cases all over Serbia to different hospitals, instead of keeping them in hospitals at Nish, where it first started, and finding out the cause. It seems that Serbia still requires more sanitary inspectors, though a great deal has been done and is being done at the present time.

Saturday, August 7, 1915.

I was taken bad again in the night, so I am again in bed. The doctor has given me something to make me sleep, so I feel a little better. They say I went on duty too soon after enteric. It does seem a shame that the Austrian prisoners from the hospital have been sent elsewhere today, they were such nice men and they do their work splendidly. The one that looked after my ward brought me a large bowl of flowers this morning, and he was always so pleased when the nurse allowed him to bring me my medicine. I have had forty-five letters in less than three weeks, people are so good in writing to me. I hear that I have more letters than any one in the camp. Mrs. Askew is staying in Belgrade, and she heard I was ill, so came in to see me. They have no work to do in their unit just now.

Mrs. Askew has had a horse given her, so she goes out riding every morning from 4.30 to 5.30. The chaplain, Mr. Sewell, comes to see me very often; his wife helps in the kitchen; they are a delightful couple. They come from Bristol; a good many people here come from the North of England. A little boy of thirteen years of age was brought in here yesterday; he has fever, was in the Serbian uniform, and is a sergeant-major, such a curious little fellow.

Monday, August 9, 1915.

This morning Mr. Sewell had a little service for one of the nurses who has had typhus and me; it is very nice having a chaplain with us. Still in bed, so feel rather dull. Mr. Winch, the head of this unit, paid me a visit this morning; then Mr. Sewell, the chaplain, came. Miss Trendle, the matron, brought me books and papers. A nurse was telling me a story that had been told her: the doctors heard a great scream, went out to see what had happened; an old woman had fallen and dislocated her patella; she would not allow any one to touch her, and they sent off for a funny old woman whom they looked upon as a witch. She came, and first put some sugar over the fractured part, then a poached egg; then a bandage was put on; then the old witch got people to hold the injured woman while she took the bad foot and pulled and pulled as hard as she could.

We hear that a lot of Austrians swam across the Danube the other day to join the Serbian Army; the Austrians were drowned; the Serbs sent a boat to rescue them, but it was too late. A few weeks ago one of the Serbs swam across and joined the Austrians.

Thursday, August 12, 1915.

This afternoon at 2 o'clock the Austrians started shelling this town. The first shell dropped two doors from this hospital, setting the place in flames; two shells struck two of the hotels. The shelling lasted about three-quarters of an hour, but our firing soon stopped them. It was from Semlin the Austrians were firing, and the guns must have been very big as the shells were a very large size; I have a piece of one. This is indeed a wicked war, so many people absolutely ruined and their homes smashed to pieces. The matron from this hospital returns to England in about ten days' time; she is having a picnic this afternoon in the Botanical Gardens.

One of our naval men has just come up here. It seems that the Austrians fired two shells on to Milanovatz; we replied by firing back four shells into one of their towns. The Austrians replied by firing back eleven shells on Belgrade; we sent back twenty-two shells into Semlin; then the house was set on fire two doors from this hospital. A man blew a big whistle for the fire alarm in the middle of the road. The doctor had me moved into one of the back wards, as this ward is in the range for firing; all the patients were removed to the back.

Friday, August 13, 1915.

We hear that twenty-two bombs fired from here destroyed a lot of houses and a lot of people in Semlin. Fires were seen blazing all round; only one man was killed here and very little damage done. The shells fired by the Austrians were from their 6-inch guns. The ward I am in is a mass of flowers today; a lot of the nurses brought them for me last night; they are all so kind to me.

Saturday, August 14, 1915.

This evening about 10 o'clock a fire broke out at the back of this hospital, about 150 yards away. It was a large brewery and was burnt to the ground. We watched it until 12 o'clock; the sparks were a sight floating along in the air. It was a chance for the Austrians to attack, as Belgrade was lighted up all round. The searchlights look lovely all along the Danube. We have Serbs, English and French here.

Sunday, August 15, 1915.

This morning the Serbians have been shelling some of the islands along the Danube.

Monday, August 16, 1915.

The Serbians and Austrians have been busy firing all the afternoon and evening. We hear that the Austrians have found out where the English guns are. They have smashed one of our English cannons; several Serbians have been wounded. The Austrians have been trying for some time to move their camp, as they want to go and help the Turks. The Serbs, as soon as any attempt is made, fire on them. The sky was lighted up with searchlights last night; this has never occurred before, and probably Zeppelins were expected. The searchlights are generally on the Danube and Save. My doctor here returned from our camp this evening, so I have had another doctor looking after me.

Wednesday, August 18, 1915.

Several of our unit came over from the camp today; they have two days' leave, so they have come over to see Belgrade. Two are staying on for a few days, as one is still feeling ill. I hear Dr. Atkinson is over at Vrynatchka Banja with one of the orderlies who has had an operation; they thought she was going to have cancer in the chest, but it is a cist. I am much better this evening.

Thursday, August 19, 1915.

We have had no more of the Austrian fireworks over here the last two days; I expect the Serbs, English and French quieted them down the other evening; we have plenty of large guns here. King Peter has a lovely palace, but it has been very much damaged. This afternoon I was allowed to go for a short walk, then I went to tea with one of the nurses who has had typhus. Nineteen of us went to her tea-party.

Friday, August 20, 1915.

Sister Barnes goes to Uskub tomorrow, so it has been arranged that she takes me with her to stay a few days before returning to Kragujevatz. We have had a nice wire from Lady Paget this afternoon, saying that she was sending to meet us. Everyone is so kind to me; the doctors will not allow me to return to the camp until I have had another change. This morning I went to the fort, as I had not been anywhere; the commandant took us all over and showed us everything.

We looked through glasses from the trenches and saw the Austrians on the other side; we could see the damage done by our shells on Semlin. We could see two monitors on the Danube; they are only allowed to move a few miles, otherwise we fire on them. We went into the trenches, but had to be careful not to be seen. We saw a large unexploded bomb; it was fortunate it had not burst; we also saw a small one which had gone right into a tree. The buildings round the forts are quite in ruins.

At 4.30 the matron had a carriage for me and let me go to see the hospital they have got for babies; so many babies had died through neglect, so they have got this "Baby Farm," as they call it. It looks on the Danube, and you can see the railway bridge that went over to Austria, which was blown up by the Serbs. We had tea with a friend of mine, Miss Bankhart, and the doctor who has been attending me; we could not stay long as the carriage was waiting for us. I forgot to say at the forts we went under a dark tunnel, which goes under the Danube and lands one in Austria; it is blocked up part-way now. I hear the other three nurses from Kragujevatz returned this evening; they came to say goodbye to me but I was up at the Baby Farm. I leave for Lady Paget's this evening.

Saturday, August 21, 1915.

Sister Barnes and I left Belgrade at 6 o'clock; our coachman was a boy of thirteen. He took us along a forbidden road to Topschaite; we had to drive furiously on account of the snipers in the hedges on the river Save which we were skirting, and only fifty miles away. The horses went at such a speed that Miss Barnes' box took a flying leap off the carriage; the Jehu turned round and gazed as if we were to get out and pick it up. We left Topschaite station at 8. We had some interesting Americans who have a camp at Nish; their camp is called "Columbia" owing to the unit being chiefly made up from the university of that name. One specially interested us as he told us that an American Jew had inoculated him for typhus, a thing that we heard in London was quite impossible. He was a Dr. Plot from New York; he is only twenty-five years of age.

We are told typhus is due to dirt, lice, and sanitary conditions, and it was introduced into Serbia by the Austrian prisoners. Among the other travellers who interested us was a man with a blue-grey hat, a khaki coat, red knickers and black top boots. He was very sorry for himself; his bull-dog had taken a slice out of his trousers. He carried a beautiful embossed sword. We arrived at Nish, which is a place that seems to be suffering from the seven plagues of Egypt, from flies, dust, dirt, smells, etc. We were told that the Serbs have brains like scrambled eggs, as they scatter their diseases all over their country. We arrived at Nish at 11 o'clock. We were taken to the rest house by the Americans. We visited the American camp, then went to the Serbian Red Cross office to get Miss Barnes' typhus medal. We left by the 8 o'clock train for Uskub, or Scoplie.

Monday, August 23, 1915.

We had a comfortable night in the train, arriving at Scoplie at 6 a.m. We saw a lot of buffalo and storks in the fields on the way. Lady Paget sent to meet us. We had breakfast and then went to bed. Lady Paget has Lord and Lady Templemore; they are the father and mother of Mr. Chichester who died a few days ago from typhoid. I shall be here about a week.

The change is doing me a lot of good here, and I am feeling quite better again and ready for work. I hope to return to the camp on Sunday evening, arriving at Kragujevatz early Tuesday morning. I have thoroughly enjoyed being here, and am quite in love with this place, it is so Eastern.

After breakfast Sister Barnes and I went to rest, had lunch and then went to the village in a carriage which was driven by Turks. We bought a lot of lovely things. This is the most ideal place in Serbia; it is like an Eastern village, and it is full of Turks, and the costumes are most picturesque. This has been a wet day; there is a large market held here every Tuesday. The train for Salonika left at 6 o'clock. I went down to the station with some of the doctors and Lady Paget; the latter was seeing Lord and Lady Templemore off. We met some of the Farmers' unit from Belgrade, who were passing through. We got home about 8 o'clock and I was sent to rest until luncheon. After lunch I went into the village to do some shopping with two of the nurses. Scoplie belonged to the Turks only two years ago; it is more Turkish than Serbian.

Wednesday, August 25, 1915.

This morning the four night nurses and I drove down to the market to do some shopping; I also went to see the park. The market here is very picturesque. To ring the church bells a man has to sit on the roof. Some of the roofs of the houses are made of biscuit tins; as long as the rain does not come in it does not matter what they use.

Thursday, August 26, 1915.

Have been to the Turkish villages again today. We went to see a chapel which is full of coffins. There was a white cloth over them and a Turkish hat, and also a stone at the top, and a lighted candle. These coffins have to be kept for 100 years; they contain the bodies of priests and Turkish kings. To advertise tailors here, one sees a large placard of an Englishman in a frock coat and a top hat. To advertise dentists they have large cases of false teeth, and they write the name of the dentist with the teeth. Turkish cemeteries are to be seen everywhere, and one sees skeletons and bones lying about the fields. The cemeteries are not railed in at all. There are *harems* all over the place; one can always tell them as the windows are barred. Most of the pathways round here are paved with old Turkish tombstones.

Friday, August 27, 1915.

We hear that Belgrade is being bombarded again, and that no private people are allowed to go there. This morning we went into the Turkish quarter, and we went over some old Turkish baths. I saw over the wards at the hospital; there are over 400 patients. Malaria is very bad here, and there have been several deaths from it. It is the malignant malaria that is so dangerous. Mr. Chichester died of typhoid and para-typhoid combined. Para-typhoid affects the nervous system. There is also another kind of typhoid, A and B, and one can be inoculated for the three.

Saturday, August 28, 1915.

This morning the night nurses and I drove over to see the melon and tobacco fields. The tobacco leaves are threaded on string and are dried on the outside of houses under the eaves; it looks so nice hanging down. After tea one of the sisters and I went for a drive by the river, and we passed thousands and thousands of troops coming from Albania. They were Albanians and Serbians; they had hundreds of horses, who were laden with ammunition and all kinds of transport on their backs. Lots of them had goats and fowls on their backs, which looked perfectly happy and quite tame. I expect all these troops were going to line the Bulgarian border, but we have not heard yet. 150,000 have passed through Scoplie the last few days. If the roofs of the small cottages get damaged they are repaired with petrol or biscuit tins.

Sunday, August 29, 1915.

We went down into the little village for a drive. On our way back we saw a quaint band and a lot of Turks and Serbs in the most lovely costumes, wrestling; it was amusing to watch them. I left Lady Paget's to catch the 7 o'clock train. Lady Paget came to see me off. Mr. Askew was on the train, so it was nice knowing some one.

Monday, August 30, 1915.

We arrived at Nish at 8 a.m. Our carriage was very full: a Serbian doctor, three Serbian officers, and a French lady who was travelling with me. The Serbians brought us a beautiful melon; they are quite different to our English ones. I am writing this at the station at Nish. My train leaves tonight for Kragujevatz at 8 o'clock. We got off comfortably. Mr. Askew went down and got me a nice sleeping-carriage, but unfortunately I had to change at 3 o'clock at Lapovo. I arrived at Kragujevatz at 6 o'clock.

Tuesday, August 31, 1915.

On arriving at the camp, Mrs. Stobart was just off to another dispensary. We have five dispensaries working now. Another is to be started on Saturday; this is the last. The chief, I hear, is to return to England in about three weeks, as her son has returned from America. Dr. May will be left in charge of this camp. Colonel Harrison came to dinner; he is the English military *attaché*. He is returning to England as his health has broken down. Very few English people can stand the climate for very long.

Wednesday, September 1, 1915.

Mrs. Stobart returned from the dispensary. Colonel Harrison came to dinner with the new English *attaché*; Colonel Harrison left directly after for England. He has left us the most beautiful gramophone.

We heard the sad news today that Nurse Berry died on arriving in England. She was a beautiful girl and a splendid nurse. She was my nurse when I first became ill, and she was taken bad a few days after we were together at Vrynatchka Banja; she was craving to get home.

Thursday, September 2, 1915.

Nothing of interest has happened today. I am not on duty, but hope to be in a day or two.

The weather is still very hot, but we have a good deal of wind; the guy ropes constantly want tightening.

Sunday, September 5, 1915.

We had service at 5.30 a.m. I helped one of the sisters get ready for Mr. Little. Several of the Scotch unit came up. Friday and Saturday I was busy doing the accounts, as my part has not been done since I left, and we have about fifty of the staff and 125 patients.

Monday, September 6, 1915.

I have been for two walks today, first with one of the doctors, and then with one of the sisters, the first walk since I was ill. This morning we went through maize fields, and on our way met several women spinning; they are always at their knitting or spinning working on the fields. Their knitting is wonderful as they make such lovely patterns with different coloured wools. We saw a man making baskets. He first gathered the willow sticks, which he put into boiling water, removed the skin, then he started his basket work. This morning I went up to the cemetery. Fancy, over 11,000 graves since November, 1914, all soldiers, and there are just plain little wooden crosses to each, and four in a grave. Dr. and Lady Finlay came over to see our camp; she came out with us on the *Saidieh*.

I got the accounts finished up to date, and in the afternoon about fifteen of us went off on two bullock wagons to get blackberries, as we have scarcely any jam left.

Mrs. Stobart had asked us at lunch who would volunteer. We took tea with us. We went about two miles but did not get any, only one of our unit who lost us, and she found a hedge covered and so managed to get a bowl full. The fields are full of maize, and amongst the maize they grow pumpkins and marrows, and large sunflowers, and up the maize stalks they grow beans. The soil is wonderfully rich. Some of our party brought a large pumpkin back with them. The peasant women are much to be admired; they do all the field work, and one will meet them driving the oxen and nursing a baby. The oxen are lovely beasts and so well cared for, but they are very slow in their movements. The hills round are lovely; the most wonderful colourings.

Tuesday, September 7, 1915.

I am not on duty yet, so this morning I have been doing a little washing and ironing. This afternoon I went for a short walk and got some lovely cape gooseberries and flowers; they are very plentiful. The Serbians make quite a nice jam out of the cape gooseberries.

Wednesday, September 8, 1915.

I went into Kragujevatz this morning to do some shopping; met Miss Vera Holmes. We bought a hat for one of the sisters going to a dispensary. You never saw such things; the hats are just like those at the sales in London for which we give 6½d. I went for a walk with Dr. Coxon, and as we were passing a vineyard such a nice woman called us in and gave us grapes and flowers. It is wonderful the richness of the soil, for when we arrived here in April there was very little on the land, and it all seems to spring up at once. We are getting short of provisions here; we managed to get some Serbian bacon, but when you want anything of this kind you find there is a long line of people outside the shop waiting for it to open, and my commissionaire goes in at the back door and buys it all up; it seems too bad. Tea is 15s. per lb.; bread, 8½d. per loaf; sugar, 1s. 6d.; butter, 7s.

Thursday, September 9, 1915.

I went to see a camp of Serbian soldiers; they had many large guns and carts full of shells which they showed us. Sixteen shells in each cart; they were 15 cc. They also had boxes full of rings of gun cotton, with powder in the centre; these they put on the top part of the shell before firing it off. There are about 200 bullocks and carts at this camp. The hood part of the ox-cart is used as a shelter for two soldiers to sleep under, and very comfortable it looks, and they only have a very few tents to pitch and quite small ones, low to the ground; one cannot stand up in them. Six men sleep in one tent. We went to see the aircraft guns and were shown how they were worked; it was most interesting.

We then went on to where the Serbs were practising firing the shells. They have high stone walls which they use as a target, and there are two or three trenches near the walls. We saw lots of bursted shells. In the afternoon we went for another walk and saw the women making wine out of plums. They pack large barrels full of plums, then fill them up with water and put some sugar in; these are left for a month or longer; then the liquor is drawn off and bottled. I wish the plums had been washed! We met some women knitting some elaborate coloured stockings; the colour is worked in after the stockings are knitted. Some of the walnuts here are almost as large as a hen's egg.

Saturday, September 11, 1915.

Today I have been in the wards taking the numbers down of all the patients. I also did some washing, then I got some lovely wild flowers and arranged them in our sitting-room. We have a gorgeous Indian tent; it is cool in the hot weather and warm in cold; it is lined inside with yellow. I have a very large tent all to myself; it would hold quite six or eight beds, so I am in luck's way. On my table I constantly find dishes of grapes, and tonight I found a dish of boiled corn—so good, I invited four of the nurses up to help eat it. The farm girls bring me all these good things, but of course I have to be careful what I eat. Five of the Second Farmers' unit have been to spend the day with us; one of them comes from St. Leonards. She has asked me to go and see her when I return to England. I also met a nurse from Holland; she knows me quite well by sight; she used to work for Dr. Stanley Turner at Battersea.

Sunday, September 12, 1915.

I have been for two short walks today. The fields are still a mass of lovely wild flowers, and the hedges full of red berries. I keep the sitting-room supplied with flowers as I am not allowed to do work, so I do all kinds of odd jobs.

Monday, September 13, 1915.

A wet day, so I wrote cards this morning and mended stockings. Letters and papers are coming very badly from home. We have seven dispensaries at work; Mrs. Stobart has just started the last one.

Tuesday, September 14, 1915.

I went for a walk with one of the sisters. We saw a large Serbian camp, then on to a gipsy village. We had crowds of little children after us; they are not used to seeing strangers about. We then saw a cemetery where some Austrian prisoners were digging up some old graves; the skulls and bones they were collecting and putting into handkerchiefs to re-bury them; it was a ghastly sight. In this cemetery they had little arched fireplaces made of brick at the head of each grave. I suppose in the cold weather when they come to wail over the grave they light a fire. I have picked up seven horseshoes, so I ought to have some good luck.

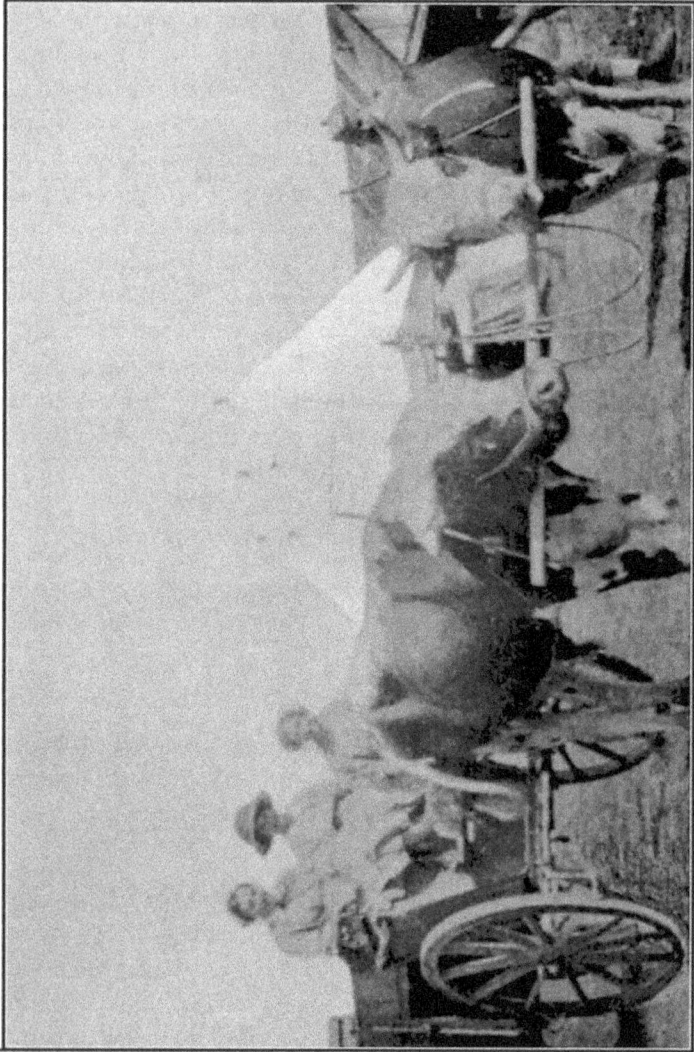

A WAGON DRAWN BY OXEN AT KRAGUJEVATZ.

Wednesday, September 15, 1915.

I was not well again today, so I stayed in bed all day. The doctors say I am not to do any work for six months in the kitchen departments; it is very annoying.

Thursday, September 16, 1915.

It seems that the peasants only have three sets of clothes to last them their life; the cloth is homespun, very strong and heavy, and a dark brown colour, most serviceable. It is trimmed with black braid.

Saturday, September 18, 1915.

Two of the sisters arrived last night from the dispensary. They have had several cases of smallpox; out of six cases in the village, two died. The peasants are the most funny people. Three days before the death of one of the smallpox patients everything was got ready for the burial. The coffin was made by friends on the premises. The girl was told, when our nurse went to feed her, not to take any more food. Before the girl was actually dead she was put in her very best clothes to be buried in; she was also laid out before the breath was out of her body. The coffin was left open until just before putting into the grave. There were no priests in the village, and the girl was buried by her friends.

Sunday, September 19, 1915.

We had service at 5.30 a.m. The priests in Serbia are not allowed to go into the church until they are married. In war time no priests are allowed to marry, so they are not able to go into the church. The priest at Natalintse went to have dinner at our dispensary. He took with him all the things that he thought they would not have, cheese and wine. They were having goose for dinner. He took this course, and then he kept stretching across the table, took a fork without asking, and kept helping himself; he had five helpings of goose. Pudding he refused, but our interpreter was sitting next to him, so he took a fork and took a taste of his pudding without asking. Five little boys keep the church in order and they ring the bell.

The priests and people think nothing of spitting on the floor of the church. I thought this habit was bad enough in the streets in England, but I find that it is worse abroad. This morning a Red Cross ambulance corps, pulled by bullock-wagons, passed this camp; they were the first to go to Malanovatz to join the first field ambulance, the Bevis unit. This afternoon I went up to see another Serbian camp, and took photographs.

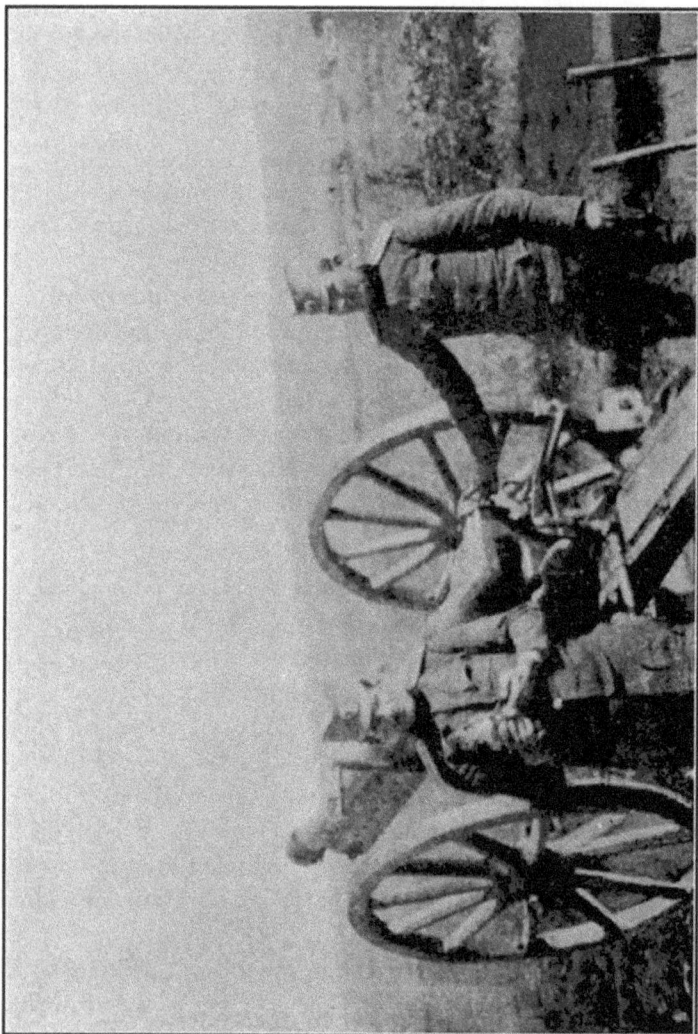

GUN CAPTURED FROM THE TURKS IN THE LAST WAR.
USED BY THE SERBS TO BRING DOWN GERMAN AEROPLANES.

Monday, September 20, 1915.

We are having lovely weather, but the nights are terribly cold, and there is a thick frost in the morning. The days are very hot. It seems that when the Austrians last year got into Belgrade they were there for thirteen days. When the Serbs drove them out, they found a freshly-made cemetery full of wooden crosses. The Serbs thought that it was strange within such a short time, and the graves were a curious shape. The Serbs turned up the soil and found about 80,000 pieces of ammunition.

Tuesday, September 21, 1915.

Mrs. Stobart, Mr. Greenhalgh, Colonel Gentnich, Mr. Little and myself motored over to Vilanovatz to see the dispensary. There is one doctor, a nurse, a cook and two orderlies; the dispensary site is very beautiful. They are doing good work and they have about 70 to 100 patients every day; they come for miles; some of them are in a terrible condition. This dispensary is fifteen miles away; the ride is lovely, the scenery being so very beautiful. The fields are looking so pretty with wild crocuses. There is only one shop in the village. *Paprica* grows very plentifully out here; the stews are quite red with it. The *paprica* is also eaten in the green state filled with meat minced.

Wednesday, September 22, 1915.

This morning one of the sisters and I went on the top of some hills to see the Serbians practising and testing some Turkish shells. It was most interesting, for they were telephoning up to the arsenal after every one that was fired, stating the distances. In the afternoon we both went up to get a shell; there were fourteen unexploded ones.

Thursday, September 23, 1915.

We have heard nothing but firing most of the day. I forgot to say that on Tuesday a message came up from the government to say that an aerial raid was expected, but they were again driven back.

Friday, September 24, 1915.

Today we hear that the Bulgarians have joined with the Austrians, and that fighting has started on the Bulgarian frontier. All along the Danube and at Belgrade the Austrians were bombarding. One hundred shells were fired.

Saturday, September 25, 1915.

Today we had a message from the Serbian Government to say that part of our unit had to go to form a hospital near the Bulgarian frontier. The Serbians have a splendid equipment ready. Twenty of this unit are going: Mrs. Stobart, Mr. Greenhalgh, two doctors, six chauffeurs, two cooks, two orderlies, and six nurses. They are taking six motors. We shall be very busy here with so many of the staff away. The doctors want me to stay a little longer to help in the wards, do the diet sheets and the accounts, and help the nurses.

Sunday, September 26, 1915.

We had two services today, one at 5 a.m., the other at 5 p.m. We are still having very hot days but the nights are cold. The wild flowers are beautiful, and there are lots of butterflies, little blues, and a dark yellow with black edge round the wings, and swallow-tail. There are scarcely any cabbage butterflies here, but there are some quite small white, like the cabbage.

Monday, September 27, 1915.

The part of our unit that was to go to the Bulgarian frontier had to be inspected today, with all their baggage. There is some difficulty in getting through to Salonika, owing to the troops going to the frontier.

Tuesday, September 28, 1915.

I hope to be back on duty in a few days. Tonight the sky was most gorgeous, quite indescribable; there were two of the most beautiful rainbows, absolutely perfect, with a sunset which illuminated the mountains all round. Moles are very plentiful here; they make a dreadful mess of all the fields. One lived under the ground-sheet in our sleeping-tent, but, poor thing, it got trodden on and we found it dead. There are a few bats; they are a tremendous size, much larger than they are in England. Grasshoppers and locusts are also plentiful. Small birds are scarce, only a few sparrows and swallows and sand–martins and larks.

The swallows have their nests right inside some of the houses on the tops of the electric light and in some of the corners. They fly about at night, catching flies, not caring for any one. We heard last night that the Scottish unit had lost one of their nurses, with typhoid; it was at Valievo. Dr. Inglis, from Kragujevatz, and the head of the Scottish women's hospital, a woman doctor, had to read the burial service. I had a lovely large bunch of hyssop given to me this morning; it is used in the churches at christenings to sprinkle the infant with holy water.

Wednesday, September 29, 1915.

Today we had a medal presented to us from King Peter. It is a coat of arms on a cross of Serbia, and is called the Cross of Charity. Two of the government officials came up to present us with them, and they gave us a testimonial of their appreciation of our services. We hear today that the Bulgarians have started fighting. I saw some of the Serbian cavalry starting for the Bulgarian frontier; they were going to Nish, then towards Pirot. The Serbs are very brave and some of them stand pain so well. One man had an operation on his spine, some broken bone removed, and he was walking about two hours after. Another man had some varicose veins removed and he was walking ten minutes after.

Thursday, September 30, 1915.

This morning at 7 o'clock we had an air raid; six German aeroplanes came over dropping thirty bombs on Kragujevatz. Most of the bombs dropped near the arsenal and at the station; they tried to get the magazine, but did not succeed. The bombs did little damage, but six people were killed and several wounded. We brought one aeroplane down; we saw quite plainly and the bombs seemed to drop right on the aeroplane—a great blaze of fire we could see—and the aeroplane fell to the ground only a few minutes' walk from this camp in the main street, just near the cathedral. It came down quite gently, and as it got to the ground there was a great crash; the men were both Germans; they were smashed to pieces. I have taken two photographs; all the woodwork was burnt away. I have several interesting pieces of the aeroplane. The Germans had their diaries on them; these of course were taken to the Government office. An officer was killed at the arsenal, so they had a military funeral for him this afternoon. The other portion of our unit may go to the front any time now; they are only waiting for orders.

Friday, October 1, 1915.

This morning at 6.45 we had another air raid. We soon cleared the camp of the patients. Three aeroplanes came over in all, and dropped about fifteen bombs on Kragujevatz. Five fell in the arsenal, but little damage was done; several fell round about the station. Several of the station men got into a truck for shelter. One shell fell just outside smashing up the pavement along the line. A piece of the shell went through the truck; no one was injured, and it was given to me afterwards. The air raid lasted about one hour. When all was over Dr. May and Dr. Berry asked me to take them to see the aircraft guns. These were about seven minutes' walk from the camp on the top of a hill; two of the Serbian camps were also near by. I knew several of the officers at the camp. On arriving we were met by some of them; they took us round and showed us the guns and the shells, explaining and describing all about them. There are three very large guns, and these took the 12 inch shells; they were of French make, and two smaller ones which were captured from the Turks in the last war.

We had only been up on the firing ground about five minutes when the signal was given that enemy aeroplanes were sighted. All men were at their posts in a second, and it was splendid to see the order and discipline.

It was no use our retiring, as it would not have been safe, so we stood by while the firing was going on. The vibration and noise were terrific; one could not see even these large shells coming out of the guns, only fire and smoke. I took a photograph while the firing was going on. Five bombs were dropped in Kragujevatz, one on our camp, which fortunately did not explode. It was only a few yards away from the night nurse's tent and mine, otherwise we should have had our poor tents in pieces. Two bombs fell on the magazine, destroying lots of our stores; three tents were burnt, but the fire was soon extinguished. Nine 7 lb. tins of marmalade were smashed to pieces; marmalade was all over the floor, windows, ceilings and walls, making the place in the most terrible mess; other stores were also spoilt; pieces of shrapnel were found in the sugar. About eighty shells were fired on the aeroplanes, and it got so hot for them that they soon fled. The air raid was over at 10, so our patients were allowed to return.

In the evening we had a farewell party, given by one of the sisters, as she was leaving for Lady Paget's hospital, and twenty of our unit were leaving for the Bulgarian frontier with Mrs. Stobart, and they were to go to Perot. They left at 10 p.m., and slept in the train all night; the train left at 7.20 in the morning. They have taken five motor ambulances, three bullock wagons, one kitchen that was captured from the Austrians by the Serbs, a few bandages and medical stores. A Serbian army was supplying all the other necessary medical stores and equipments for "The Flying Field Hospital." I was to have gone, but owing to having had typhoid was not allowed. It was arranged that the doctors, nurses, cooks and orderlies should change over every month, so that all could get a variety of work.

Saturday, October 2, 1915.

Another telephone message arrived at 7 a.m., to say that three aeroplanes had crossed the frontier. We got breakfast over at 5.30 and the camp was cleared of all the patients, and then we left ourselves. It is interesting to see all the townspeople going out miles into the country for safety. Fortunately the wind got up and the flyers had to return, but they managed to drop their fifteen bombs on another town close by. On our return home to the camp we went by the guns, and I was introduced to the man who brought down the aeroplane on Thursday, September 30. It was the Turkish aircraft gun he was using, quite a small one. We expect air raids every day now; this means breakfast at 5.30. We are clearing this hospital of the old patients, and are getting ready for the fresh wounded, and it will not take us long to be straight.

We can do nothing much in the mornings now, so we work hard all afternoon. The arsenal is also closed in the mornings.

Sunday, October 3, 1915.

It has been too cloudy and too windy for an air raid today, so we have had a day of rest. Pontoon bridges have been passing most of the afternoon on the road by our camp. I expect these are going to the Bulgarian frontier.

A very young student at a village near here was full of mischief, and for a lark he poured a pot of red paint into the holy water. The priest at the early service looked up, and found that all his congregation had red crosses on their foreheads. The priest told us this story, and the boy got into great trouble over it.

The name of the aeroplane that was brought down at Kragujevatz was the "Albatross." The younger German killed was an engineer twenty-six years of age.

Pieces of aeroplane were found at Ratcher, but nothing else. Another aeroplane was seen to turn over outside a small village, but has not been found.

Monday, October 4, 1915.

The camp was cleared about 7 o'clock, as we received a message that six aeroplanes had been sighted over the frontier; they were prevented from getting to Kragujevatz. The Germans say they will smash up Kragujevatz, also the railway line. A very little damage has been done considering.

We had a card from the other part of our unit which left for Perot, saying that they had arrived safely, and that they liked their position; they were on the top of a hill, and looked down on the enemy.

Tuesday, October 5, 1915.

Two aeroplanes flew over Lapovo, dropped three bombs on the line, but no damage was done. We cleared our camp as on previous days but nothing happened.

Wednesday, October 6, 1915.

We are about ready for the fresh wounded; we have put up one or two fresh marquees, which hold each about twenty-six beds. We have seventy-two tents in all, and a number in reserve if required. We have long buildings when the weather gets cold, which have been built during the summer by the Austrian prisoners; these were intended for cholera, but fortunately we did not get this disease in Serbia, so the buildings have been promised us by the government for wards for our patients during the winter months. They are very long low build-ings and would hold about thirty or forty beds; there were about six buildings in all.

On one occasion, in our ward, a patient who was on light diet, was found to have a parcel under his pillow. This parcel was found to contain a little roasted pig, from which he had been helping himself to small pieces. His relations had been to visit him that afternoon and had given it to him, regardless of whether it was a suitable present or not. Pigs in this country are cooked when they are quite tiny, and a leg is only sufficient for one person's meal. Lambs are also killed and cooked about the same age, and it is really difficult to find any meat on the bones after they are roasted. The Serbs do not consider meat good when it is fully grown, excepting oxen, and beef in Serbia is one of the worst classes of meat, probably on account of their being used for labour. Milk is scarce owing to the cows being used for transport.

They have an extraordinary one-stringed instrument which they will play for the whole of the day; crowds of people will sit round listening; this was most trying when the patients got hold of it in the wards, very monotonous and trying, and some of the singing is also very weird, being only on one or two notes, but on the whole they are the most musical people. In the cathedrals the singing is perfectly lovely, such well trained voices.

We hear that the Germans started shelling Belgrade at 3 a.m.; it lasted for many hours. We had a thick fog at night, which reminded one of London, being equally dense but not so yellow.

Thursday, October 7, 1915.

Still a thick fog, and we hear that Belgrade is still being bombarded. The English and French troops have been expected for some time to help the poor Serbs, and we are told that Nish and many other towns are decorated in their honour.

I understand that the bombardment of Belgrade has not been quite so severe today, but all English missions have been told to leave. The Germans have landed in three places. They crossed the Save in boats and by pontoon bridges; there were about 3,000 of them. It was a misty night, and they thought they would not be noticed. The Serbs allowed them to cross, and then took 2,000 prisoners. The pontoon bridges and boats were sunk; then they had a hand-to-hand fight in the streets, knives being principally used, and we heard that even the women joined in. Many bodies were floating in the Danube and the Save; we heard that two of our marines were killed and several wounded.

This afternoon we went over the wounded Allies' hospital at Kragujevatz with one of the sisters. In one ward there was a brigand who was wounded; he had told the nurses that that was his profession. We also saw an Austrian who was an artist, and he had obtained in the hospital several orders for his pictures, for which he made the sum of 10s. We also saw a German who had had both his legs amputated; he was allowed to make baskets, and was selling them.

This evening one of the doctors consented to my leaving, as having an appointment in England I had only another two or three weeks leave of absence and as we heard it might be rather difficult later on to get away. I was asked to look after an orderly from the second Farmers' unit, who had just recovered from typhoid; she would not have been able to do any work for some weeks so it was decided she should return to England in my care.

Friday, October 8, 1915.

I was busy packing most of the morning, then I did up the accounts and the diet sheets for the wards, finishing up this part of my work. In the afternoon one of the sisters and I went to the arsenal and I was presented with a medal of King Peter. We also saw many of the treasures which were taken off the German aeroplane which was brought down. They showed us an orange printed paper with full instructions on. It was of course in German and it said that they had to come to Kragujevatz and drop four bombs.

It was very painful saying goodbye to my kitchen staff, principally Austrian prisoners who had done such good work. When they first came they said, "No pay, therefore no work." I replied, "No work, therefore no food," and they quickly fell in with my views, which they never resented but really worked well. The commissionaire came up to say goodbye with his daughter, and brought from his wife two cooked chickens for our journey, a dozen eggs, walnuts, apples and jam. I packed these up, then went in to dinner. When I returned I found my parcels had been unpacked by the dogs from the farm near by; the chickens had gone, the eggs eaten, and bits of shell all over the floor of my tent. Eggs when boiled hard out here the white will often be found soft no matter how long one boils it. Also the apples and the nuts scattered about; my tent was a sight to behold, but fortunately we had other things provided for the journey.

At 9 o'clock fifteen wounded men were brought in from Belgrade. They were in the most terrible condition, and they described to us the most awful slaughter that had taken place there.

At 10 o'clock one of the Government officials came up to say goodbye, and to bring my pass on the railway as far as the Greek frontier, and also gave me some sweets.

At 11.30 the carriage came to take us to the station. The train was leaving at 12 o'clock. A terrible night, pouring with rain, and we all got wet through before starting. We had a comfortable journey as far as Lapovo, where we arrived at 2 a.m. Here we had to change, and were supposed to get a train on in an hour's time, but waited about till 5 o'clock, and were then told that there would not be a train on till noon. We piled our luggage up and went to our dispensary, which is on the line. We found the windows open and the door unlocked and everyone in bed. They had left it like this as they were expecting the doctor from Nish, who had gone to fetch fresh supplies of stores. We took off our boots and lay down on the beds in the ward until 7 o'clock, then we had breakfast and took it in turns to go back to the station to take charge of the luggage. It was a pitiful sight while in the station, watching the train loads of refugees coming in from Belgrade. Many of the women were crying as they related their sad experiences to the people on the platform. Also train loads of wounded were coming in; many had been to our dispensary on the Thursday to have their wounds dressed before going on to a permanent hospital.

We were told that 6,000 or 7,000 shells had been fired in Belgrade, and that many places were on fire.

At 11 o'clock a train came in from Belgrade, and I heard several voices calling to me, and I found there were some of Admiral Troubridge's unit on the train, and three or four of the first Farmers' unit. They all looked very ill and were covered with mud. They had left Belgrade at 6 o'clock the night before, and had had to walk many miles before they could get the train, and had left everything behind them, only having the clothes they stood up in. They had only had bread to eat and were almost famished, so I told them to come and get into our carriage, as we could give them some of the food we had for our journey. I then went to the guard and asked where this train was going to, and he replied "to Nish"; but there was only a cattle truck for us, so we all got into it, and as it was very doubtful about our getting a train at 12 o'clock we thought it better to go on. We gave them all a good meal of tongue and beef sandwiches, bread and cheese and apples and lemonade, and they were indeed thankful, poor things! for they had gone through a terrible time. They told us many sad stories of our brave Serbians, who ran into the hospitals, had their wounds dressed, and then went back to fight.

All the patients in the hospitals who were suffering from bronchitis, pneumonia, and consumption, and many other diseases, put on their clothes and went to the trenches. They also told us that the American hospital was staying on, so all their luggage was sent to this hospital for safety; later on the American hospital was seen in flames. The members of these units got out of the train at Chupria, to join Admiral Troubridge. We heard that the English batteries, with the exception of one, had been quieted at Belgrade. At Chupria many wounded soldiers got into our truck. They were going to the hospital at Nish, we to the rest station which belonged to Sir Ralph and Lady Paget, and it was for the use of the different English units that were coming to Serbia. We arrived at 9.30, and as we were very tired we went to bed at once.

Sunday, October 10, 1915.

We had breakfast at 7.30, then went to see Sir Ralph Paget, then to the bank, which fortunately we found open, then to the Serbian Red Cross.

Several other members of different units arrived from Belgrade during the day.

At 2.30 an enemy aeroplane came over Nish. No bombs were dropped, so they had come to spy. Three French aeroplanes went after it and drove it away; they also fired on it with the aircraft guns. We heard that one of the trains from Belgrade had been fired at by the Germans and that twenty-five civilians had been killed. We had a service at the rest house at 5 o'clock. Two aeroplanes had arrived during the afternoon and were going on to Kragujevatz.

We left by the 8.30 p.m. train for Salonika.

Monday, October 11, 1915.

It was a lovely day and most interesting journey. All along there are camps, wire entanglements and trenches. Some of the camps are amongst the trees and can scarcely be seen, as they are made of sticks and mud. The sentry guards also along the line have curious dug-outs, to which they go down by steps. The haystacks, instead of being on the ground as in England, are fixed up in trees, like huge beehives, as the ground gets so swampy. The Serbs and the Albanians look most picturesque. These must have been the regiments I saw coming along when I was staying at Uskub. We have just seen a wolf chasing a young deer; they passed close by the train. It seems dreadful to leave this glorious country with its brilliant sunshine and bright colours, until we see all the horrors that are going on so near to us.

We arrived at Uskub at 7 o'clock; had breakfast at the station, and a few minutes before our train arrived 170 Bulgarian prisoners had been brought in. They were tied together in batches by ropes. I saw one or two of the nurses from Lady Paget's on the platform; they had been to see some friends off. Our train left again at 7.25; then we passed through wonderful gorges; this of course would make the fighting very difficult.

Our next stop was the frontier Ghevghili (?). Most of the passengers' luggage was examined; it was also weighed, and we had to pay on ours.

We arrived at Salonika at 8.30 p.m. We found the station full of Greek soldiers; many of them were on the ground asleep. We had to leave our large luggage for the night, then we took a carriage and went to the Hotel Olympus, where we had wired for rooms. We saw many of our English and French troops as we drove down; this of course cheered us up. We heard there were 25,000 French and 11,000 English, and that they had been detained by the Greeks, as they were expected in Serbia some days before.

On arriving at the hotel we made ourselves tidy, went down to dinner, found the room full of English and French; several of them gave us a hearty welcome as there were no English women in Salonika. One officer told us that an American, sitting at their table had insisted on it that we were Americans, and what a great deal the Americans had been doing in Serbia, and the point had been argued, so there was great excitement to know what nationality we were, and the English officers were delighted to find they were right.

We are all hoping that the Greeks will join us, and that they will all be going up to Serbia in a day or so.

Tuesday, October 12, 1915.

Two English officers invited us out to tea to the *café* near, and were much interested in hearing all our experiences in Serbia. In the evening we went to a cinema.

Wednesday, October 13, 1915.

We had to go and have our passports inspected by the English, French, and Italian consuls; we got some money changed and did some shopping.

The Turkish markets are very interesting and the salesmen very amusing, and bargaining is very necessary as they begin by asking often more than double the amount they are prepared to take.

The Greek shops are very fine, full of beautiful things, and the fashions quite up to date. We have a nice little Greek lady staying here from Athens; she told us it was a known fact that the Germans had lost over three million men. She also told us that seven French officers had escaped from Stuttgart; they were let out of prison as they bribed the man who was looking after them. They walked all the way from Stuttgart through Switzerland to France, having been given sufficient food for their journey, a compass and a map, and advised not to speak to any one on the way. They said they never met a man all the way through Germany; women were armed outside forts, railways and along roads; every man had gone to fight.

Thursday, October 14, 1915.

There are eight battleships in the harbour, French and English. The Greeks are mobilised, and are ready to join whichever side they think the best. They have copied the English in their uniform.

A Turkish aeroplane passed over today. Our boat, the *Sydney*, has arrived in the harbour, so we went to choose our berths.

About forty boats arrived today with English, French, and Greek troops. We went to watch the horses and mules being unloaded at the docks; there are more mules than horses; they find them much hardier.

Friday, October 15, 1915.

We had an interesting day; one of the doctors from Lady Paget's came to see me, then the captain from the *Abbassieh,* who had brought out some of the units and knew the three sisters who were with me. He invited us to lunch on his ship; he had brought in troops from the Dardanelles, and was doing transport work. He told us that he had brought 1,300 and that he had only sufficient life boats for 300. In Salonika we had the Dorsets, the Norfolks, the Herefords, Royal West Kent, Royal Engineers, the Army Service Corps, and the Royal Army Medical Corps, and several other regiments that were going up to Serbia.

The captain asked what boat I had come out on to Serbia. When I said "the *Saidieh,*" he said, "Why, the chief officer is now on my boat, as the *Saidieh* was torpedoed some time ago"; and he sent for him to see us. It was very pleasant meeting again and hearing his story; he was made captain of another boat, but it had been so much damaged with shell fire that it could not be used.

Saturday, October 16, 1915.

In the afternoon the commander from the battleship H.M.S. *Albion* came to have tea with us, and invited us to tea on his ship the following day.

We heard today that some of the French troops had gone up to the Bulgarian frontier; we also heard that Perot had been taken by the Bulgarians, and that the line between Nish and Uskub had been blown up.

Martial law is in force here, and pickets are all along the front. The English, French, and Greek officers all had to salute each other.

Sunday, October 17, 1915.

This morning we went over two old Greek temples, Demetrius and St. George; they were taken by the Turks and turned into mosques. The Turks had whitewashed all over the mosaic and marble pillars; fortunately the whitewash is crumbling away, and one can see the mosaic through.

A story is told that one of the large panels of marble is supposed to bleed when anything serious is going to happen; it is a kind of grey-red, very lovely, and the blood trickles through the cracks. The priest in Demetrius was standing with a cross and a piece of *bosaliac,* known to us as *hyssop.* The Greek soldiers were going up to him, kissing the cross, and then he sprinkled their heads with holy water with the *bosaliac.*

We went to see the wonderful old bridge that Hadrian, the Roman Emperor, built.

In the afternoon we went to H.M.S. *Albion* to tea; it is a very fine ship, and of course of great interest to us. It has been damaged many times with shell fire; we went all over and it was most interesting.

Lady Paget arrived here last evening, and five of the sisters from Admiral Troubridge's unit, as they had been staying the night with her at Uskub. Two of them were returning to England with us.

Monday, October 18, 1915.

We hear that the *Sydney* sails tomorrow at 4 o'clock, so we made our preparations for leaving.

We have seen crowds of refugees coming into the town today, many of them sleeping on the doorsteps, huddled up in the corners. One poor man died on the road, and I expect many others will not survive as they had walked so many miles.

Tuesday, October 19, 1915.

We got our luggage on our boat the *Sydney* early, then we took a small boat out to the hospital ship, the *Grantully Castle*, London, as the military doctor said the matron would so much like to see us. On arriving we were received by the matron and the English chaplain; we were taken all over the ship; it was beautifully fitted up, and they had every convenience. There were three of our naval men from Belgrade, two of whom had been wounded, and the other one was threatened with appendicitis. Forty English soldiers had been taken on board the night before, suffering from illnesses of different kinds. The nine nurses were Australians, the matron English. We were invited to lunch, but could not spare the time, as we had to get back early to the hotel on account of leaving in the afternoon.

We left the hotel at 3.30 and at once went on board. One of the doctors from Lady Paget's hospital is with us, two of the nurses from Admiral Troubridge's unit, six of the Scottish nurses from the women's hospital, Valievo, two French doctors, and an English lady from Bulgaria who had been teaching there for the last six years, also the military *attaché* from Bulgaria, a naval member of Parliament who was carrying dispatches, also Brigadier General Koe, who was engaged in transport work.

We left Solonika at 5 o'clock. This boat is quite nice and beautifully clean, very different from the one we came out in. It is a French boat belonging to the Maritime Line. We had a good passage as far as Lemnos, where we arrived at 7 p.m. General Koe got off here.

Wednesday, October 20, 1915.

Lemnos is a barren-looking place, mountainous all round, no trees, and it is covered with the English and French camps. There is a new hospital being built at the water's edge. There is no fresh water, and experts have been sent from England to sink artesian wells. The water had to be taken out in tanks. One lady at Marseilles sent out ship-loads of soda water for the soldiers. The harbour is full of battleships, chiefly French, and there are several hospital ships, also many transports. The largest ship is the *Aquitania* from Liverpool, with four large funnels. Mines and nets are all round us; at several points of the island guns are fixed; we could hear firing this afternoon, and we were told that at Imbros one could see the shells bursting at the Dardanelles. We stayed at Lemnos eight hours; it is a lovely day and very calm.

Thursday, October 21, 1915.

We arrived at Piraeus at 6 a.m., landed at 8, then took the train to Athens, and went straight to Cook's office and wrote letters to friends staying here, arranging to return for any answers. We then took a carriage and went to the museum; the statuary is very fine and beautiful. We returned to Cook's and found a letter from our Greek friends, inviting us to luncheon at 1 o'clock. We had an hour and a half more to spare, so took a carriage and went to the Acropolis. It is indeed wonderful the view of Athens from the top, most beautiful. We thoroughly enjoyed this sight; the trees all along are most interesting—avenues of pepper trees, date palms, aloes and cactus; we also saw a few orange trees. We then went to our friend's house at 1 o'clock.

There were three married sisters and their children, and an English girl, governess to the children. After luncheon they took us sight-seeing, first to the Polytechnic Institute, founded in 1837 by some wealthy Greek, and containing memoirs of the Greek War of Independence, portraits and native costumes, and the clothes of the Greek king who was shot at Salonika. A tomb has been erected on the pavement there where he was shot, and a chapel is to be built near. The pistol that shot him was in the case with the clothes. We also saw many flags that the Greeks had captured in many different wars, a sword of Lord Byron's, and his portrait and visiting card.

After leaving here we took the carriage and drove round the principal streets, then went to the Keremakos market, where there are wonderful tombs containing the remains of three people in each; the bones are visible, and the statue of the bull. We then went down the oldest streets, and to the ancient Church Eglise de Capnicarea. We saw the temple, the bank, the general post office and the theatre; had tea at a *café* and took the train back to the port, and arrived on the boat in time for dinner. Another lovely night; I slept on deck. I forgot to mention we passed, on Wednesday, some burning rocks; the chief officer told us they are set on fire by oil by the shepherds, to watch their flocks by night.

Friday, October 22, 1915.

We did not leave Athens until 8.30 this morning. We were held up much longer than we expected. An aeroplane followed our boat for a little way, but it was a Greek one, so we had nothing to fear. At 3 p.m. we had quite an excitement; a message was sent to the ship to say we had to go into the Island of Milos for orders; submarines had been seen round the neighbourhood. We got into Milos and found five French battleships, submarine destroyers. One of the maritime ships was in the harbour that had been torpedoed two weeks ago. The island is very picturesque; the houses are built in the Turkish style. We remained in the harbour for about two hours.

We have a submarine destroyer escorting us, also another ship was with us, so we feel quite safe. Written notices were sent round to each passenger with instructions what to do in case we were struck. The captain had an anxious voyage from here on, keeping watch all the time. We kept going out of our course and the destroyer and our boat were constantly signalling to each other. We had to come round by Crete instead of Cape Matapan. The wind has risen and it is very rough; most of the people are ill. We had a bad night, continuous thunderstorms and heavy rain. The boat is rolling as well as pitching.

Saturday, October 23, 1915.

It still continues very rough and very few passengers are visible. Nothing exciting has happened; our two escorts are still in front of us.

Sunday, October 24, 1915.

This morning a large steamer signalled to our destroyer, so it left us for two or three hours and then returned. In the night it was exchanged for another one. We were told that they had to be very careful along this route, as nine boats were torpedoed in one week; naturally we were all more or less anxious, looking down into the cold water. I much dreaded the risk we ran as I should much prefer to be shot or shelled to being drowned. We heard that we reach Malta in the evening, but owing to our having to go so much out of our course we did not arrive until the following morning at 6 a.m. It was an anxious night; neither the captain nor the chief officer appeared for dinner; no end of men were on the watch for enemy submarines; it seems that there are many in the Mediterranean just now, and we were told that this is the worst danger zone at present. The Germans have a specially large new one here which is doing a lot of damage.

It has been very rough all night, and the boat had to slacken speed as we were not allowed to enter Malta before 6 a.m. I met a very interesting English lady from Constantinople on board this morning. She has lived there for forty years. Her husband is a doctor. She had three sons—two solicitors, the third an invalid. He suffers from fits. The youngest son's name was down on the list to be sent to Gallipoli with the English and French prisoners, whom the Turks were sending from Constantinople, in the hope that this would prevent our troops from bombarding Gallipoli. This poor mother was so distressed, and pleaded so hard to the Turkish officials that they consented that her son should be released. She then made another plea for her husband to be allowed to leave the country, and he left for Malta. Then she procured the release of her delicate son, and he also joined his father, and now she herself is on her way to join them. The other two sons were not allowed to leave; they are being kindly treated, but have come down to breaking stones. I felt very sorry for her, but admired her courage and cheerfulness in such distressing circumstances. All her valuables from her lovely home she sent to the Turkish bank, but of course has no hope of seeing them again; they are sure to be confiscated.

Fifty or more of our men were sent to Gallipoli from Constantinople, so that should the place be bombarded they would be the first to fall; but the English and French threatened the Turks with other reprisals, and they were withdrawn. They left the ship and spent five days in a mosque, where they had to rough it terribly, though the officials were very kind to them, and on their return to Constantinople gave them a good dinner. Everybody out here speaks so well of the Turks, and all those we have met seem so very sorry that they are fighting against the English, and they said it would be their ruin joining the Germans, their great dread being the loss of Constantinople. Three little birds are following our boat, often coming on board; one is a robin, but the other two we do not know. We had several cats on board and were much afraid for the safety of the birds. Two sparrow-hawks also pursued them.

Monday, October 25, 1915.

We were allowed to land at Malta at 8 a.m. As we only had three hours on land we took a carriage, only 1 *fr.*80 the hour, and drove all round. The carriages are different from ours, so picturesque, and the Maltese women, with their curious headgear, are very fascinating. We went first to the gardens to see flowers and palms, which were look-ing lovely, then to the Church of St. John's, where a service was taking place, so we remained a little time. We saw the governor's palace, then the Chapel of Bones, formerly attached to the hospital. Over 2,000 skulls are shown, and the remaining framework of the body is most artistically arranged, but very gruesome. We had not time to enter the museum as we had to do a little shopping before returning to the boat. We sailed at 11.30, still very rough, and we could not keep a straight course; our escort was with us.

There were three suspicious characters on board, and we hear they had been locked up.

Tuesday, October 26, 1915.

Still very rough, and most of the passengers have had to retire; those who were able to remain played bridge.

We have no butter for tea, only biscuits and dry bread; this was not such a hardship to me as to some of the other passengers. We had had no butter in Serbia for more than three months as butter cost there 7*s.* per pound, and as we could only obtain such small quantities, even at that price, it was not worth buying for our large unit.

Wednesday, October 27, 1915.

We had a bad thunderstorm today, and the sea is still very rough. Nothing of any importance happened.

Thursday, October 28, 1915.

We arrived at Marseilles at 8 a.m., for which we were all truly thankful, as it is not much pleasure to be facing such dangers as we had done.

At the Customs our luggage was most carefully searched, even the leaves of our Bibles and other books being turned over. We were all much amused and wondered if we should be searched next. This I believe happened to some of the women, but not any of our party.

We had our passports seen, and also paid a visit to the police station to obtain a pass to Boulogne. This took up most of the day, and we remained two nights in Marseilles. There is an Indian camp, as they come here to be climatised before going to the front. It was interesting seeing them about the town.

Saturday, October 30, 1915.

We left at 7 p.m., and on our arrival at Boulogne found the times had been altered, and our boat did not leave until the next day at 3 p.m.

Monday, November 1, 1915.

When we got on to the quay a hospital train came along, and we were told our king was in it, and his boat left just before ours, so we felt quite safe—and not at all sorry when we arrived once more in England.

The Retreat from Serbia through Montenegro and Albania

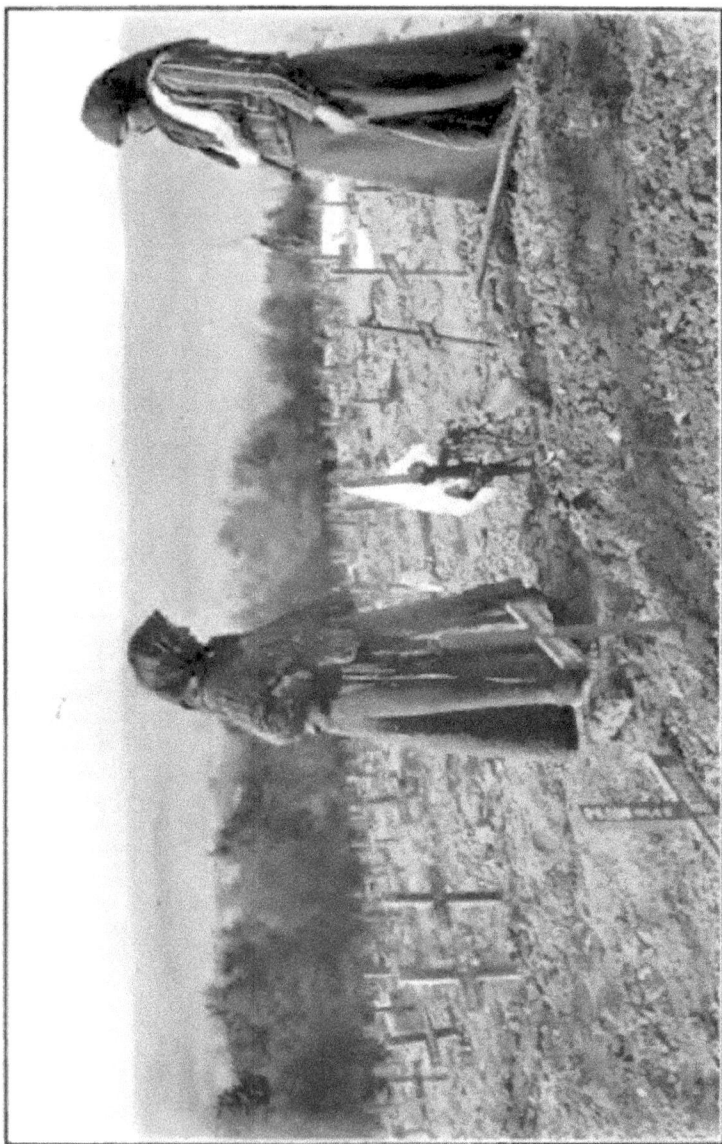

"FROM THEIR BLOOD WILL SPRING FLOWERS FOR SOME FAR OFF GENERATION." — NJEGOS.

Contents

Introduction

In July, 1915, I went to Serbia as a member of the 3rd Serbian Relief Unit (sent out by the Serbian belief Fund Committee) to work at one of the village dispensaries which were then being started by Mrs. Stobart in outlying villages within a radius of some thirty miles from her Field Hospital at Kragujevatz.

The outward journey was by sea to Salonika, and thence by rail to Kragujevatz. After spending a short time at the Field Hospital, I began my village work; this lasted till early October, when it was interrupted by the invasion of Serbia by the Austro-German and Bulgarian Armies. The three weeks which followed the renewal of fighting were spent at the Kragujevatz Field Hospital, where wounded soldiers were brought in from the Belgrade area. Early in November, when the fighting in that district had stopped and the road lay open to the invaders, Kragujevatz was evacuated. Then for seven weeks I was on the road with Serbian soldiers from Kragujevatz to the coast of Albania and finally reached London on December 23rd.

In this short period of time I had thus seen Serbia under three different aspects: first, life in the village when the land was in a state of comparative peace; again, when the country was invaded on three sides and the Serbs were fighting for their lives; and yet again, when, after defeat, they were retreating before the on-coming foe.

In the following pages I have tried to reflect as I saw it a picture from each of these three chapters of Serbia during those eventful months and have added a note on Serbian history.

In the final adjustments of this terrible war may my country do all within its power to secure justice for the liberty-loving people of this Eastern land! O. M. A.

41 Russell Square, London, W.C.
August, 1916.

To

THE SERBIAN PEOPLE

PART 1

The Village of Vitanovatz

It fell to my lot to be stationed at Vitanovatz, a small village a little less than thirty miles south from Kragujevatz and some seven miles north from Kraljevo.

Three women were on the staff—Dr. McMillan and Sister Collins for the dispensary, and myself as housekeeper. There were also David Boone, an English lad, as chauffeur; Joseph, a Macedonian, who was to act as interpreter for the patients; and Sam, an Austrian prisoner of war, to assist in the general household duties. Both the latter were placed at our disposal by the Serbian Government.

We travelled out one day from Kragujevatz in a red car which belonged to the Serbs, and a big motor lorry from the Arsenal brought the stores, tents and other equipment. The road was heavy and difficult and the lorry writhed and snorted on the hills as it pressed slowly forward like some sentient creature quivering in its struggle for breath: at points it seemed as if nothing could prevent it from breaking in two, so great was the strain. The swift red car ran ahead from point to point and then waited for long intervals for the lorry. We started our new home in a field adjoining the village.

The field was hilly and sloped towards the road; there were several fine old trees in it and it was bounded by hedges that later in the autumn were laden with bright-hued berries. Our living-tents were pitched on the ridge of the field, and the dispensary tent at the bottom of the slope quite near the road. A notice was put up, in Serbian, to say exactly who and what we were and to invite anyone who wished for medical aid to come to us. The village was chosen because the road running through it led to the little town of Kraljevo, and many peasants in the course of a week went by with their produce.

News of our coming spread quickly and the peasants flocked to the dispensary in large numbers after the first few days; many with real maladies, for whom much was done and many cures effected, but others came too who were perfectly well but affected illness from sheer curiosity to see what we and our camp looked like. We were "an event" in the village, many had seen no one exactly like us before, and certainly we were the first people from Western Europe who had come to settle in the village.

So the peasants came to find out how we talked, how we dressed, what we looked like and what we had to eat. The excuse for coming would be to see the doctor. This formality over, they would walk round the dispensary tent and inspect it in detail, then they would walk slowly up the field to our private quarters. It never surprised us to enter our mess tent and find a group of peasant women discussing its arrangements or to enter our sleeping quarters and find a similar group deeply interested in our camp beds or the shape of our garments; or still another group round our fire lifting the lids of our pots and pans to find out what we had for dinner.

A bright yellow fisherman's oilskin of mine, brought from England, attracted much attention, and when wearing it, whether in the camp, in the village or in the market town, peasants who had not seen it before would come straight towards me as though they had been attracted by a magnet; sometimes two or three people would take hold of it at the same time, apparently forgetful that someone was inside it, feel it and pronounce it "*dobro*" (good). The village people too seemed to know where it was kept on fine days. Even the *presednik* (the magistrate of the village) openly admired it and told me laughingly that he would steal it should he have the opportunity. Other members of the staff had equally good mackintoshes and of far greater value, but these excited no interest and we attributed the attractiveness of mine to its colour—bright yellow.

But if the Serbians found us interesting because different from themselves, we certainly found them interesting, and for the same reason. Being chiefly an agricultural people they have a different civilisation and—apart from the Catholic, which we have in common—a different religion: most are members of the Greek Church and others are Mahommedans, and not only have they another language but another alphabet, the *Kyrillic*, based on the Greek instead of the Latin characters. Then, too, there is a fortnight's difference in time between their calendar and ours. Two other points of difference we noticed among the peasants—a nod of the head we found meant "No," whilst a shake of the head meant "Yes," and that the women, who are great knitters, invariably commence a stocking at the toe instead of the top. The Serbs belong to the East of Europe and are therefore quite other than ourselves and have much of the reserve of the Oriental. At first it was the differences that roused our interest; later we not only admired but found the Serbian character lovable.

We not only helped the peasants with medical advice, but with clothing when there was need. Our assistance was accepted quite naturally and was looked upon as the gift of one friendly nation to another, and they in their turn were equally ready to help us. The Serbs are a kind, generous natured people and are always ready to give. For the smallest services rendered them we were always repaid; gifts of fruit, nuts, eggs, vegetables, live pigs and chickens, knitted gloves, coloured waist belts, amongst other things, were showered upon us. Things they themselves had made or had grown on their little farms. Sometimes we did not like to take these gifts, as the homes from which they came seemed to contain so little, but to refuse would have hurt their feelings. They are a sensitive people and to give is so much a part of their nature that we always accepted. A peasant woman from a neighbouring village who occasionally washed clothes for us, always gave us a big rosy apple each when we paid the bill. One day a peasant entered our tent whilst we were at dinner; he went round the table and gave each of us three walnuts, then walked away.

Many patients came journeys, which took several days, in bullock waggons over the hills and along what appeared almost impassable roads. They slept in the waggons and brought food enough to last till their return. On arrival the oxen would be unyoked, then people and animals would sit down together near the waggons with their meal spread on the grass, and a fine day would see our field dotted with these ox waggon groups, the oxen eating hay or stalks of maize. Maize is a great food in Serbia for both man and beast. Animals and people have many things in common, and a great intimacy exists between them; the animals too seem very human.

An ox we met once on the road from Kraljevo was very surprised and frightened on seeing our motorcar. For a time he stood quite still and gazed, his eyes growing ever larger and rounder, then dashed for safety to the side of a woman who stood with a distaff in her hand a little way down the bank by the roadside—just as a child might have run to its mother's side for protection—and from this point of safety watched the car pass.

Animals, and people too, take life at a contemplative pace, both seem to live ever in an atmosphere of dignified leisure and are seldom in a hurry. When asked to do anything the peasants would always reply "*sutra*" (tomorrow)—and tomorrow never comes. We too after a little while when asked to do things said "*sutra*" with the ease and fluency of the native—possibly it was the climate, for we too began to feel that anytime would do. Peasants who came long journeys would wait quite patiently their turn to see the doctor and it appeared not to matter whether their turn came today or "*sutra*." Our staff—or rather its western element—were the only people in a hurry and who bustled round and fussed over things. Soon we began to feel that all this haste was not only undignified but almost indecent, and had we stayed a little longer, just as we had learned to say "*sutra*," we too might have learned fresh values for things and realised there was no need to hurry and bustle—eternity was before us.

The Serbs, men and women, are fine in stature and have very handsome dark eyes. They begin to look old at a very early age. Often have we been shocked to find that patients whom we had thought long past middle age, were quite young men. Possibly it is the effect of their hard outdoor life. The men dress in brown home-spun garments trimmed with black braid and white or unbleached under-garments; in summer the under-garment is worn outside. The outer garment is sometimes very ragged and bits, large or small, of the underwear may stick out at many points, but this never affects the easy manners or bearing of the Serb. We often remarked that he possessed a soul above rags and other surroundings. Certainly there is no element of snobbishness in him. Silk sashes of varied and brilliant colours are worn by the men under their brown jackets, and the women are fond of gay embroidery on the fronts of their bodices; their skirts are very full and rather sombre in colour.

The foot gear of both men and women is a kind of sandal called "*opanki*." In wet weather the women take off their *opanki* and walk down the muddy roads and across the fields with bare feet. A narrow leather strap run round the top of the *opanki* acts as a drawstring and keeps it close to the foot. The end of this strap is taken round and round the leg and fastened with a metal hook in the stocking just below the knee. The top of the stocking is a favourite place for carrying a big knife. Often the Serb—who, in days of peace, is a gay fellow—will fix a little bouquet of flowers, a rose or a geranium at the point where the strap hooks into the stocking, another bright flower will decorate the front of his cap which is worn a little on one side of the head, and yet another will be carried in the barrel end of his rifle. A lover of flowers is the Serb, and music is a part of his nature; he takes life easily, and perhaps a little indolently. Often were we fascinated by his gay appearance as he sat on the grass in our camp. And yet this same man would, if danger threatened, rise to attention on the instant and be ready if need be to face death on the spot.

Such a man was Svertomir (a Serbian orderly added later to our staff) who we all agreed was a bad housemaid but a good soldier. He never cared for washing the saucepans (*lonats*) after supper and would ask with a smile if they could be left till the next day, "*Sestra! lonats peri sutra pet sat?*" (Sister, saucepans clean tomorrow at five o'clock) and when morning came often they were not ready for cooking the breakfast. Yet when garbed in his soldier jacket (a little small for his stalwart form) with knife in belt or stocking, and shouldering his rifle and fixed bayonet, he was transformed and could be trusted in any emergency. He accompanied us later in our "*trek*" down to San Giovanni di Medua, unfailing in kindness and helpfulness, bearing privation without a murmur, after a hard day's journey taking his turn cheerfully as guard at night. We owe Svertomir much. We left him on the Albanian coast, far from the little home in Kraljevo where his mother lives.

The Serbian women work on their little farms (the peasants own their land) and when not actually engaged in this work are always seen with knitting needles or a distaff in their hands. They knit thick heavy stockings and gloves for their menfolk and embroider them with gay floral designs in vivid hues—often one saw a man wearing bright yellow woollen gloves with green or red roses worked on the backs.

There were two inns in the village quite near each other, both double-fronted buildings, and each had a wide roomy veranda on the ground floor, hung with creepers and other plants, extending along the full frontage. A few steps led up from the road to the veranda, which had to be crossed in each case to enter the inn. Seated round the tables on the veranda were always groups of villagers discussing the latest war news with wayfarers. The inns resembled our old-fashioned country inns in the days before railroads. Roads in Serbia are not easy for travellers, and distances between towns are great. Rooms in the inns we found were primitive but clean and comfortable, floors were uncarpeted. Travellers often brought their own food, it did not matter whether they bought it or not at the inn.

There was good stabling for the animals. In many of the Serbian villages inn fires were lighted in small recesses in the walls, some five feet or so from the floor, over these water and coffee would be heated in tiny tin or copper pots with long handles. At one inn we had two rooms, of which we had the keys, for storage purposes. Here we kept our stocks of medicines and provisions and other things which it was necessary to keep dry.

One large common room in both inns was used permanently by Austrian prisoners. In wet weather their meals were taken there. Other prisoners occupied a loft over some stables. The Austrian prisoners made a new road to our camp; they worked in the village and in the fields, and being thus healthily employed by their captors had perhaps as good a time as any prisoners of war. The *presednik*—or magistrate—of our village let them take the apples and pears from his orchard when they were working for him, "although," he said with a smile, "they do not deserve them." He, the *presednik*, was kind to us and looked after our wants. He it was who kept us supplied with wood for our fires. When our supply ran short we used to send him word and he would send Austrian prisoners to cut down a few trees, which were then drawn up in ox waggons into our camp, accompanied by Austrian prisoners to unload and cut them into the requisite lengths.

Many of the peasants never chopped their wood, but placed the end of a tree across the hearth—a square hearth often in the middle of the room—and lighted it; all that was necessary to replenish the fire was to push the tree as it burnt away a little further across the hearth. Often there were no chimneys and the smoke went off in any direction it pleased. These fires in the middle of the room were very fascinating to the outsider. One house near us had such a fire and in passing, just after dark, we could see through the open door a family of eight seated round it with the light flickering over their faces and the children with their little hands stretched out for warmth outlined against the flames. The rest of the room was in shadow and darkness. Another house with a square hearth and space for quite a large tree was often visited by us, as a consumptive lad lay dying there and his parents were anxious to obtain medical advice from every possible source. "Will he get better?" was always their question. "If there is a chance we will give him only the food that is good for him; but if he must die, then he must have whatever he wishes." He was a soldier in the Balkan War and contracted the illness in Albania, where he had been sent to fight.

The *presednik* sent water for general use to us from the river in large barrels, drawn up to the camp by oxen; our drinking water came from a spring near the pope's (the minister's) garden. Great interest was shown by the *presednik*, as by the peasants, in what we had to eat, for in addition to the things bought in the district, we had stores sent out from England. A new kind of bean or pea was at once commented upon, whilst the canned foods and our ways of cooking caused much serious reflection. The *presednik* would often call just before meal times, and he too would lift the lids of our pots and pans to see what was inside. Taking out his knife—all Serbs carry large knives—he would cut a piece from anything that was new to him, eat it, his face wearing a serious expression the while, and finally would make his pronouncement in judicial tones.

Sometimes we would ask him to share our meal, and if we then offered him anything with which he was familiar he would wave it aside with a lordly dignified sweep of his arm and say he could get it "*svaki dan*" (every day) and so would have none of it; if, on the other hand, he could not get it "*svaki dan*" he would eat heartily. He was an intelligent man and took a keen interest in everything that concerned the area under his jurisdiction.

Presedniks are elected every three years; they are the chief men of their areas and can adjudicate in all questions of land and other property up to a given value. Our *presednik* was eager to establish a school in Vitanovatz that all the children, he said, might learn to read and write. One day he took us to a neighbouring village—also in his jurisdiction—and showed us over a school in which he, as a boy, had been one of the first scholars. He wanted both a church and a school at Vitanovatz. "Which," he asked us, "should come first?"—and when we said the school he was delighted because it fitted with his own ideas. He was a deeply religious man, but the school, he said, meant so much to the children, and churches were more frequently accessible.

"Besides," he said, "God is everywhere." He took us too one day to a village church on a special feast day and we saw the churchyard almost filled with peasants from the neighbourhood who had brought food to place on the graves of their dead; those who brought the food gave it to all who came, and ate of it themselves. The ceremony is called "*datja*," and is a very ancient custom amongst the country people. Those who partook of the food thought whilst doing so of the suffering the dead had endured, and the souls of the dead were thus benefited. The peasants went in single file through the church and each received a blessing as they passed the altar and kissed the hand of the "Pope"—a cold, lifeless-looking hand which he extended. He seemed no longer human, but inanimate, and might have been a decorative section of the altar. Later, this time in the open air, standing at the end of a table, the "Pope" blessed the representatives of families and villages who came forward with bowed uncovered heads.

In this village we called on the peasant woman who washed our clothes and were welcomed by her with whole-hearted hospitality; she brought us jam and water, which it is the custom to offer. A little tray is handed with a dish of jam (the fruit is kept whole in the preserving), two receptacles for spoons, and several glasses of cold water. The etiquette of the ceremony is to take a whole fruit, put the spoon back in the receptacle for used spoons and then drink some cold water. At first the ceremony, though simple, is a little puzzling. During the walk back to our own village we talked with the *presednik* about the government of the village, his election to office and his Committee of Council. We told him about the villages in England.

A pleasant weekly event was my visit to the *presednik's* office to pay for eggs, milk and garden produce bought through him from the villagers. At first we bought direct from the peasants, but found it difficult to refuse to buy when the articles had been brought long distances, and consequently got overstocked with goods. The *presednik* arranged that the main orders should be given through him, and he would distribute these as fairly as possible amongst the villagers. In these weekly finance visits all the formalities of such a proceeding were duly observed. The *presednik* sat at his table with his clerk by his side as the various items on the lists were checked. No element of frivolity ever entered into these proceedings—it was business.

But business done, all matters under the sun would be chatted over. There was always a kindly tolerance in the *presednik's* attitude. Later, during the retreat from Kragujevatz, when relays of our unit passed through Vitanovatz, he would take no payment for the eggs, milk and other provisions he gave them. Once he was very eager to talk about a quotation from a London newspaper which had appeared that day in a Serbian journal. Many speeches were being made in London about Serbia. The Lord Mayor of London—who, by the way, we translated as the " *Presednik*" of London—had referred to British friendship with Serbia; another important personage had made a speech in which he spoke of Serbia as the "Gateway to Constantinople" and had said that the main interest would be transferred from the Western to the Eastern front and that all the great issues of the war would be fought out on Serbian soil and how the Allies would come to Serbia's aid.

The *presednik's* face flushed with pride as he spoke of the part his country would play in that great decisive combat that would bring victory to the Allies and peace to the world. "What matters it now," he said, "if Bulgaria is in league with our enemies? Have we not already, and singlehanded, driven the Austrians and Germans from our land? Now with the British and French to aid us, nothing is beyond achievement!" His country now is in alien hands and he himself in exile.

Kraljevo market was always a delight to us. Often we did the journey there and back on foot, sometimes we drove—or rather jolted—in the wicker post carriage with hay for a seat. A feature of the market was the small display of goods. The peasants brought their produce in very small quantities and they seemed quite indifferent whether one bought the goods or not. They shewed their goods when asked, but though they were always quite polite they did so with a "it does not matter if you do not buy" attitude. One day a woman was sitting on the ground with a basket of apples near her and talking to a group of other women; we wanted apples, but we could not make up our minds for some time as to whether she had brought the apples to market to sell or whether she had herself bought them and was about to take them home.

The market place with its shady trees, crowds of peasants garbed in many colours—yellow predominating in their headgear—groups, of oxen sitting or standing near their waggons placidly watching the scene, quantities of walnuts at every turn spread in front of the shops on pieces of matting, was always full of interest. We made many acquaintances in the town, amongst these the Director of the Agricultural College, who visited our camp, and the apothecary who helped us in several difficulties. We also made the acquaintance of a Russian doctor and a Russian engineer. They too visited our camp. Before they came they made us promise to give them an English pudding.

When we asked "What sort of pudding?" they said "Oh! any kind, only it must be quite English." We gave them their wish, but as they came in the afternoon and had to leave early to get back before nightfall they had boiled apple pudding for afternoon tea. At the Café de Paris, in the Market Place, we got delicious coffee, and at the *café* opposite we stabled our horse and carriage when we drove to market, and took a room there to which our purchases, as we made them, could be sent and kept ready for our return.

Road scenes on the homeward journey were varied. All sorts of people and animals were there; many little wicker carriages like the one we drove in; peasant women in their "*opanki*" (sandals) and full skirts, their heads tied up in black or yellow kerchiefs, with a basket on each arm, were on horseback riding astride on very high saddles; families of pigs spreading themselves across the road and often stopping to take a meal considerably handicapped our speed. A Serbian horse is apparently only trained to walk or gallop—it never trots, and so any obstacle at once reduced us to walking pace. Then the slow, easy-going teams of oxen which, with their drivers, were always ready to be startled by anything new on the road (such as ourselves), would suddenly run their waggons at strange angles up or down the banks by the roadside; often too a number of young colts running by the side of their mothers would frisk in and out and across the track of the other animals, people and conveyances with all the irresponsible movement of youth.

Fruit, vegetables, eggs, etc., in plenty could always be got from the market or from the people in our own village; white bread too could be obtained, not so white as the English bread, but better in quality. Maize grows everywhere in abundance and, growing on the ground between the thick maize stalks, were yellow and green pumpkins. Plums, a small deep purple variety, grow too in profusion, and from these "*rakya*" is distilled.

The land is rich and has a wild aspect, though much of it is cultivated, for the peasant never overdoes it and always knows what to leave to nature. An air of freedom too is everywhere: one can wander at will and is never confronted by "Trespassers will be prosecuted" or even a "Keep off the grass!" Our neighbourhood was rich in wild flowers and berries. There were many birds. Herons and magpies were quite common—the latter as numerous as sparrows are at home. Good cheese could be got of two kinds—one "*sir*," a hard cream cheese, and the other "*kymak*," of a soft crumbly nature. Butter we never saw, and "*pekmes*," a jam made from plums, was one of our stock substitutes, and as we could not have "bread and butter," we had " bread and jam," " bread and marmalade," or "bread and treacle" for a change.

After we had lived about two days in the village we thought it but fit and proper to call on the pope (minister) and his family. We reasoned that as we had come to live in his village and could thus be looked upon as residents, and as we got our drinking water from the spring near his garden—so it was our duty, as well as a pleasure, to make the call. We did not know much Serbian; certainly we knew the names of the different parts of the body and a little about aches and pains, but we had nothing in our vocabulary that would make "polite" conversation. As the pope's family did not speak English, and any language they knew other than their own we did not understand, and any language we knew other than our own they did not understand, and as we were the visitors—the aggressors, so to speak—nothing remained but for us to talk Serbian. We felt our country's reputation was at stake and that it was up to us to make good.

A brilliant inspiration seized us, and we dived into our pockets for our sixpenny *Easy Serbian* books, turned rapidly over the pages to find material to build sentences, and after a few seconds asked cheerfully but perhaps rather breathlessly, "Have you any dogs?" When they told us, we followed up by asking, "Have you a horse?" Then, "Have you oxen?" and so worked steadily on through the list of the animals. When this was exhausted we said " Long live Serbia," and came away. A firm friendship, however, began that afternoon between our camp and the pope's household. Jam and water was offered us again at the pope's, followed about fifteen minutes later by some Turkish coffee served in very small cups, very sweet and nearly half grounds. The white floor boards in the pope's house were spotless. The walls too were white and many coloured samplers and tapestries hung on them. Bunches of dried thistle plants stood on the tables and served as holders for photographs.

The children of the village were little wild things, and at first—though filled with curiosity—would have nothing to do with us. At last after being much smiled at by us they were tamed, and a chorus of little voices would greet us in a village street with "*Dobar dan,*" "*Dobro veche,*" or "*Laku notch*" (good day, good morning, good night). They liked sugar and we would often give them a piece each as we came from the village shop. Serbian children are very serious and look like grown people cut down—perhaps the dress gives this effect. As the children get older they become less serious and look younger.

A little boy about six years old looked after cows in our field. He was so small and wore such a large wide brimmed hat and a pair of very mannish grown up trousers, that we named him the "cowherd." He was very shy, and when we made advances would have nothing to do with us; like a little wild animal he would never let us get nearer than a given distance—and we wanted so much to be friends. Once we offered a sweet, but he would not come near enough to take it; we turned away, but knowing that his bird like glance was on us left the sweet in the broken bark of a tree. A few seconds later the sweet was gone.

Fate, however, ordained that we should be friends. Sitting at tea in our mess tent one afternoon we heard piercing cries. At once we ran out and found our little "cowherd" in tears. He now not only let us approach him, but he himself came towards us, and from his sob broken utterances we discovered that he had lost a cow. Two cows only stood where three should stand. The little cowherd's attention had been so completely absorbed in watching our tents that he had not noticed the straying of the third. All ended happily; his mother came on the scene and the other cow was found, we having helped in the search.

Facing the inns at Vitanovatz was the well; this was walled round the top to the height of four feet or so, and high above this a wooden arm was balanced across a support. To one end of the arm a cord was attached, and the bucket to the other. The village possessed two shops; from the first we bought milk, from the second, the chief shop, we bought kerosene, bacon (*slanina*) which was always all fat (bacon with even the faintest streak of lean we never saw), pots for cooking and tobacco for the orderlies. The shop-keeper and his family would smile a welcome and let us wander round the shop to search for the things we wanted but of which we did not know the names, whilst other customers would try to aid us by talking Serbian and giving us walnuts or other things to eat from their baskets or pockets.

Dorothy Picton and Dorothy Brindley, of the Kragujevatz staff, came to us, one to regain strength after an attack of fever, and the other to rest after strenuous work. The former had a small bell tent to herself which we called the "detached villa," and the latter shared a tent with Sister Collins and myself, which we named the "tenement." On many windy or wet nights have the occupants of this tenement got up from their beds, gone the round of the tents to slacken or tighten the guide ropes, or to chase away the dogs who came to help themselves to the camp provisions. There were many dogs in the neighbourhood and all seemed semi-wild. At nightfall they would creep stealthily through the grass and round our tents in the search for stray pieces of food. The *presednik* lent us an oak cupboard so that we could keep food in safety at night. For weeks the dogs came, we could hear them but never see them, as they always made off by the time we came on the scene.

One night a big noise made by the falling pots and pans came from our kitchen tent. We went quickly and this time made a "catch." It was a puppy so young that it could scarcely stand and swayed from side to side as it walked. It then persisted in coming into our tent and cried in a small squeaking voice. Its mother would not be far off, we felt, and so retired to bed. A little later when all was still she came and took the puppy away.

In speaking of Kragujevatz we would sometimes abbreviate the name to "Krag'." Joseph, our interpreter, was amused. "Why do you say 'Krag'?" he asked, "the Serbs will never understand what you mean."

"Oh!" we replied, "it is shorter, easier, and life is not long enough to pronounce every name in full."

Whereupon Joseph answered, "In England, when you speak of Manchester do you call it 'Man'?" Still he was rather impressed with "Krag," and we heard him use it several times afterwards. It pleased us to make Joseph laugh because he was a pessimist and wore a dismal expression, and if there was a black side to anything he never by any chance missed it. Later, after a short time spent in the camp he became happier, and his face, instead of running from north to south, began to run east and west. He was the only person in the camp who ever carried an umbrella. Joseph—like the *presednik*—is an exile.

Four Josephs were connected with the camp—the interpreter and three Austrian prisoners who came up from the village to help us. Simply to shout "Joseph," would have produced four when only one was needed, so we added numbers to their names. The interpreter— Joseph *jedan* (one) remained simply "Joseph," the others were Joseph *dva* (two), Joseph *tre* (three) and Joseph *chetiree* (four). Much merriment, which they appreciated, was caused by the use of these new surnames. Two of the Josephs got mixed one day before they were numbered. Joseph *dva* had a severe cough and was asked to go to the dispensary tent for treatment. About the time he was due Joseph *chetiree* appeared with a message; before he could deliver this he was seized and in spite of his protests, so the story goes, had his chest examined before the mistake was discovered.

Joseph *dva* and Joseph *chetiree* were great friends and liked to work together. They took a real interest in our camp and worked hard for its smooth running. They must have come from orderly homes, for they liked to see the insides of all the pots and pans polished, and they washed our overalls and cleaned our boots without being asked to do so. They both came from a village near Prague. As twilight fell, and after a hard day's work as Joseph *dva* sat by the fire and watched the pots boil for supper, his gaze would be fixed in the direction of Prague and a feeling of home-sickness would come over him. Sometimes we would sit by the fire too and he would tell us about his home and about his capture—for nearly a year he had been a prisoner in the hands of the Serbs. The Austrians never liked the Serbian shoes they had to wear when their own wore out. Joseph *dva*, one evening by the fire, when the longing for home was strong within him, suddenly took off his *opanki* and threw them away amongst the firewood, said he had done with them and would go to Prague. Then laughter came to his aid and he picked up the *opanki*.

The first Saturday that we were in Vitanovatz we were startled by a strange sound of wailing which increased as the evening wore on, and it echoed and re-echoed amongst the hills till the air seemed filled with cries. It came from the women in the churchyards, we learned, who were offering food and flowers on the graves of their dead. This wild chant was a prayer of intercession sent by them to heaven. Each week this was repeated and carried on far into the night. Black flags—a sign of recent bereavement—would hang over the door or gateway of many houses, together often with articles of clothing worn by the dead member of the family. At many points on the roads we came across stones to mark a grave, or erected in memory of those who had fallen in battle away from home. One such stone on the road to Kraljevo was in memory of Serbian soldiers who had died in Albania. Little clusters of graves would confront one at unexpected places on the hillsides.

One day an ox waggon came into our camp bearing a dead child. The child had suffered from diphtheria. Its father was killed in fighting and the mother was busy on the farm, so the grandfather and the dead child's small brother came with the waggon—a day's journey over the hills. When they entered our field there was only a little waxen figure stretched out at the bottom of the waggon, with a lighted candle in one hand. Another day a man was brought to our camp in a bullock waggon. When chopping wood the axe had slipped and he had cut his foot, he was very weak from loss of blood. We placed a bedstead, from our own tents, in a corner of the dispensary which we curtained off, and kept the patient until he was sufficiently strong to bear the journey to a hospital in Kraljevo for convalescence.

All this time there were rumours of renewed fighting. We heard of the possible rising of the Bulgars on the one frontier, and of the massing of the Austro-German troops on the other. The Serbs were under no illusion as to their position, they knew that the renewal of fighting was near. They knew that so soon as Russia suffered a set-back at Austrian hands then their own turn would come. Rumours swept daily over our village as clouds sweep across the sky. We heard often of the coming of the British and French troops. One day we heard that the Allies were at such a place and we turned up our maps to find out how long it would take them to come north—but they never came. Then we heard that it was a mistake and they were somewhere else—again we believed it and again they never came.

Then we heard from members of another unit how, farther south, the stations had been decorated with flowers, the school children out and the place *en fête* to welcome the Allies as they entered Serbia, and that they did not come. Then we heard that the reason our men were so long in coming was because they had disembarked at a Montenegrin port and the journey across the mountains would necessarily be slow, and again we found it was all a mistake and that they had never been in Serbia.

About this time we read a leading article in *Le Journal des Balkans*—a small sheet published in French. The writer spoke of the failure of the Allies to reach Serbia and said it was now too late and, though no bitterness was expressed, there was a deep note of disappointment and a sense of coming tragedy. The article ended in predicting a second Belgium. Newspapers from home reached us but irregularly; we never got a paper less than fourteen days old, so we knew but little of the English view of the situation, and never caught the events up in the English papers before the lines of communication were cut.

One day all the bright boys in our village—as bright and bonny as any lads in any other country—were called up and taken by the *presednik* to Kragujevatz and to Kraljevo, and life in our village was saddened. Many soldiers passed through our village in the night. Joseph spent every moment he could get away from the dispensary to waylay people who came through the village from Kragujevatz or Kraljevo to get news.

About this time—the beginning of October—it was necessary for me to make a journey to Kragujevatz for fresh stores and medicines. These journeys were taken by us in turn and were always something of an adventure for until the moment of starting came we did not know what kind of conveyance we should get. To go by railway meant walking to Kraljevo for a train at noon, then spending many hours of the night at Lapovo junction and reaching Kragujevatz in the early hours of next morning. So the road journey was preferred. When we wanted to go we told the *presednik* and he would stop the first conveyance bound for the right direction. All he had to do, we said, was to stand in the middle of the village street, hold up a spread-out hand and command a conveyance to halt, as a policeman does at home to stop the traffic.

A conveyance might not come for several days, but we had to be ready to start at any moment after we had given notice. It was like a lottery and there was always a good deal of speculation as to what kind of vehicle it would be our luck to draw. The vehicle that fell to my lot was a rather small-sized charabanc drawn by two little grey horses, their long tails almost swept the ground and they were either very old or very tired, for their action much more resembled standing still than movement. The pace was so slow that one could almost count ten during one revolution of the wheels. The driver, the only occupant besides myself, was very old, or very tired too, and he continuously cracked his whip in the air, and *"Ide, ide"* (go, go) came mechanically from his lips; but the grey horses, probably as used to the sound as they were to that of the wheels behind them, made not the slightest effort to quicken their pace. Still it was pleasant to amble, for the hedges and fields were clothed in rich autumn tints and the rivers and streams were full and rushed swiftly down their courses.

The halfway stage was reached as darkness fell and here a halt for the night was made—the road being much too heavy to continue the journey after dark. During supper in the common room of the inn an American doctor came to see me. Someone had told him a "Frenchwoman" had arrived and he was a little surprised to find a Britisher. He was working in the district and spent a great part of his time, with an interpreter, in travelling on horseback to the isolated peasants' houses. The landlady of the inn was kind and anxious for me to be comfortable. Later she shewed me to my room, which seemed a combination of bedroom and store-room. There were two beds in the room, both with clean coverlets, but which probably had not been recently used, for when the beds were opened, mice ran from under the pillows. A bottle of cold water was brought for washing purposes; this had to be taken outdoors where the contents could be poured over one's face and hands, for there was no basin. An inn opposite had its frontage covered with coloured paintings in which heroic Serbian figures were depicted slaying the Turkish foe.

By half-past five the next morning we were again on the road to Kragujevatz and it was as though we had continued through the night, for again "*Ide, ide*" came from the driver's lips, again the whip cracked and again the grey horses—in spite of their supper, night's rest and breakfast, made not the slightest quickening in their pace. As the early mists rolled away, again the countryside in all the gorgeous hues of its autumn covering was revealed. Gipsies (*Tziganes*) too were seen in groups with their horses and flocks by the roadside—the horses appearing as wild and untamed as their owners. These nomadic people added beauty and interest to the roads by the richness of their complexions, flashing eyes and the wealth of colour and variety in their clothing.

Suddenly the quiet road became astir, guns were heard, the gipsies hurried to and fro, motor cars full of soldiers appeared, it seemed, from nowhere, and the road was filled with many people. My driver, shewing his first sign of real life, quickly turned the grey horses round and made them face the hedge. Then Taubes could be seen coming towards us driven out of Kragujevatz, all movement subsided and everybody stood still in the roadway watching and waiting, and the report of the guns continued. The Taubes disappeared and in a few minutes all was normal again. The remainder of my journey was completed in an arsenal car which soon outdistanced the sad little grey horses.

Happily no bombs had been dropped from the Taubes on Kragujevatz. The first wounded men were, however, coming in to our hospital from the Belgrade area. Many were brought on stretchers, but some of the less seriously wounded walked from the station, gaunt, dusty, tired men with arms and heads bandaged and clothing mud-covered and bloody. Some of them were in uniform, others in their peasant dress of brown home-spun. Amongst the many wounded men we saw, then and through all the terrible time that followed, uniform did not seem to matter, and their clothing was often a patchwork of the soldier's and civilian's garb.

Thus at last had rumour become reality—the Bulgars had risen and the Austrians and Germans, who had so long menaced our peace, were besieging Belgrade. David Boone drove me back to Vitanovatz in one of our cars, and we carried with us instructions to close the dispensary. This was to be done without delay—no matter what we were doing or how many patients we had all work for civilians had to stop and we were to go back to our hospital at Kragujevatz—nearer the scene of fighting—and be ready to do our part in all the terrible eventualities that the renewal of fighting would bring.

Part 2

The Renewal of Fighting

The Serbian soldier is brave. In courage no one can surpass him, he is absolutely fearless and holds death in contempt—not that he wants to die more than anyone else does before his allotted time. He loves life and brightness and gaiety, but with duty before him and death in the way he will go straight on not only without flinching, but without even a change of expression. He knows how to die—it is more than courage, it reaches sublimity.

It is one thing to fight if success or the possibility of success can be seen, but it is quite another thing to fight if at the end of one's best efforts there is nothing but swift and sure defeat. Against the Austrian and German army alone a longer, and perhaps successful, stand could have been made—for the memory of the last fight nearly a year before was still vivid in the mind of the Serbs when they hurled the invader back from Belgrade, and the Bulgars alone could have been easily overthrown; but successfully to repel invasion on three sides was impossible, and the Serbians knew that they were outnumbered.

Kragujevatz was the important military centre, the big arsenal was there, and all that it contained had to be taken away or rendered useless before the enemy's arrival. The government, the army—comprising all men and boys between eighteen and fifty—and all the lads between fifteen and eighteen who would supply the army for the next few years, in fact all who were liable to be taken as prisoners of war, were ordered away. There were too the Austrian prisoners—between forty and fifty thousand—to be cleared from the country.

While all this was being done and in order that others might get safely away and the retreat be carried out in an orderly manner and without panic, it was necessary to hold the invader, and so a living sacrifice was made. If courage alone could have won the fight victory would have been with the Serbs.

Austrian prisoners paid fine tribute to the Serb's qualities as a soldier—"There is no finer soldier," they said. This too is how they accounted for the large number of Austrian prisoners in Serbia, whilst their own country, so much larger and stronger, had captured so few Serbs. We who were there know something of the fight the Serbs put up because the results in human wreckage came through our hands in our hospital at Kragujevatz. We got back to Kragujevatz in time to assist in the transference of the hospital from the tents to a permanent building erected by the Serbian Government by Austrian prisoners' labour during the summer months.

The building covered a great deal of ground and consisted of long wards on the ground floor only. The removal, which had to be done quickly as the wounded men were being brought in, was made very difficult by the deep mud and heavy rains. Our staff was small, as one section of our unit was away with Mrs. Stobart with the army on the Bulgarian frontier, and another was at Lapovo, the railway junction between Kragujevatz and Belgrade. Dr. May was the chief of the Kragujevatz section. My work lay now in the hospital wards, to fetch and carry and render any services the nurses might require from me.

For three weeks wounded soldiers were brought to us in trainloads and in bullock waggon loads. Men with ghastly wounds, with only the first rough dressing put on on the battlefield, exhausted from hunger and want of sleep; night and day they came. It was as though the long line of ox waggons would never cease. At first a fair amount of comfort could be provided, clean linen and beds. Later they came in such large numbers we had to make mattresses from bags and pieces of sacking, which we filled with fibre. Mattresses were taken from the men who had both mattress and bedstead for those who had neither. Hay, straw and blankets were spread on the floor and some men had to remain on the stretchers on which they were brought.

Others were laid on the bare floor of the barely finished ward. Men of all ages were there—some quite young lads like those who had left our village of Vitanovatz. One laddie, badly wounded, smiled up from the straw where he was placed and said "*Laku notch*" (goodnight). A man near him with eyes protruding and inflamed craved for darkness and sleep.

Scarcely had these men come into hospital and barely, it seemed, before they had had time for food or rest, the *narednik* (sergeant major) would come through the wards and give out the order that all who could walk must leave at a given time. No matter what their wounds, so long as they could stand and their heads were sufficiently clear to enable them to keep their balance, they had to go, and men who needed sleep and rest stepped once again into their dusty, dirty, blood-stained clothing to take to the road, the road that was to lead them, though they did not know it then, right down to the Albanian coast, to put as great a distance as they could between themselves and the invader. Taking up their bundles, and with a *"Fala, sestra"* (thank you, sister) and a *"Sretan put"* (good luck) from us they would go their way. The road leading south-west out of Kragujevatz was, in addition to all the other people, lined with these bandaged and broken men. There were but few conveyances for them.

But in spite of all the sad surroundings both patients and staff were cheerful and little things constantly happened to cause merriment and laughter. Life is made up of a curious jumble of joys and sorrows, of pleasures and pains. Some men came back one day after they had left and found their beds occupied by others; they took it as a joke and settled themselves in the corners, and by the sides of their old beds on the floor. One patient, a Serbian sergeant, would wear his cap in bed. He always pulled the clothes up close round his chin and ears, leaving only his face visible; his eyes black and sparkling could be seen the length of the ward and he wore a dark fearsome moustache like the German emperor's. The sister-in-charge told him she would have nothing to do with him because she was sure he was the *Kaiser.*

This caused much amusement, and as long as he remained in the ward he was known as "the *Kaiser.*" Much fun was caused when we tried one evening, taking him to be a patient, to prevent an Austrian orderly from going out to get his supper. Relatives of the wounded men who lived near would stay for hours in the ward and bring baskets of cooked food, which they would spread on the bed and share with the patient.

Just as the Serb can face death so can he also bear pain. He makes light of wounds and will not stay in bed if he can possibly get up. The doctors and nurses used laughingly to say that, what with the quick coming and going of patients and the constant getting out of bed of the others, how hard it was to make the man in bed correspond with the chart hanging over his head. The Serb is strong and, possibly because he has always lived much in the open air, his wounds are quick to heal. One man who had one side of his face severely damaged and one eye destroyed, sat up in bed shortly after his wounds were dressed and smoked a cigarette.

A bright lad of about eighteen had an arm so badly damaged that the doctor wished to amputate it. The boy refused. A foreign doctor must have the patient's permission. Fearing for the lad's life the doctor said to the interpreter, "Tell him that if he does not have it off he will die." The lad without a change of expression said, "Then I will die!"

The orderlies in our hospital as in others were Austrian prisoners, and they worked wholeheartedly during this terrible time—doing all the disagreeable tasks for the patients, fetching and carrying for them, humouring their every whim, never losing their tempers and doing all with infinite kindness: the wounded Serbs could not have received kindlier treatment had their own relatives attended them. It seemed, as one watched them, incredible that the two countries were at war with each other. There were some wounded Austrians and Germans in the hospital.

An Austrian who was convalescent would run about the ward (wearing his cap and wrapped in a strangely cut dressing gown from our linen store) and spend much time waiting on the others when the orderlies were busy; he made everyone happy. At his request a bandage winder was fitted to the bottom rail of his bed and he insisted on winding the bandages when the dressings were done. Another Austrian prisoner sawed wood to make fracture beds, and another came into the ward and filed a ring from the badly damaged hand of a wounded Serb. During this time six new nurses arrived. Their train, the last up from Salonika, was bombed. They came at a time when their services were most urgently needed and also in time to lose their new equipment and share the adventures of the "trek."

All this time a low rumbling noise could be heard; it was from a never-ending line of ox waggons, in Government transport service, that passed along the road in front of the hospital each day from sunrise to sunset. Another sound too, loud and imperative in tone, could be heard; this was from the guns of the enemy and daily grew nearer. When the wounded soldiers were dying in the ward, when nothing could be done to save them, and only the presence of someone was necessary to watch and administer any little comfort, it often fell to my lot to stay with them till the end came. Death, always sad, seemed hard and cruel in these cases. These victims in a war that they themselves had had no part in making were dying as strangers among strangers (with no one present familiar with their home, their friends or their past life) in a busy hospital near the fighting line, where all the energies of doctors, nurses and orderlies were taken up with others whose lives might yet be saved, and almost it seemed before the breath was gone from their bodies, they were removed for burial because the beds were urgently needed for others.

Fighting ceased and the road lay open before the invader. All that was useful to the enemy had gone from Kragujevatz. Orders then came for us to leave; the hospital was cleared as far as could be and handed over to the care of Greek doctors. Austrian orderlies were taken away and replaced by Serbs. We were sent off in small groups at different times with ox waggons which contained food stores, tents and general hospital equipment. The last group to leave (apart from our chief, Dr. May, and the secretary, Miss McGlade, who left a few hours later with Dr. Curcin, the Chief of the Foreign Missions for the Serbian Government) contained three of us who were together at Vitanovatz.

Our orders were to press on quickly to Rashka, choose a site for a fresh hospital and be ready for the rest of the unit when they came up with the ox waggons, tents and hospital stores. To enable us to carry out our orders we travelled in a motor car and thus overtook the others. That it was the beginning of our journey home we did not know, as it was expected that further on the Serbs would make another stand against the invaders. We left after the destruction of the railway, after the military authorities had gone and about eighteen hours before the Austrians were timed to enter Kragujevatz.

PART 3

The Retreat

The road from Kragujevatz to Rashka lay through Vitanovatz—where we overtook other members of the unit—and Kraljevo, now filled with refugees from Belgrade; and then began a long climb to the village of Ushtsche. But, despite travelling in a motor car placed at our disposal by the French Sanitary Department, the journey was slow. Serbian roads were obviously never intended for quick travelling. One difficulty was to get the four wheels of our vehicle on the same level at the same time; one wheel always would be in a hole and have to be lifted out by main force. Another cause of delay was the waiting until such time as we could persuade the driver of an ox waggon to unyoke his oxen, harness them to our car and haul it out of the mud in which it had sunk to its axles. This took a long time, as no driver was very willing or pleased to stop and in consequence lose his place in the apparently unending line of waggons.

Inside the car were five of us: Dr. McMillan, Sister Price, Dorothy Brindley, Milan, the interpreter, and myself; outside were three: the chauffeur (a Frenchman), Johanovitch (a Montenegrin from the Kragujevatz camp) on the box seat, and Droog (a Serbian mechanic) on the step. Inside, too, we had an assortment of bundles, including bedding, bread, hard-boiled eggs, a cooked ham, a lantern, a teapot, a hatchet, top boots and a hammer. Periodically we were all, with the baggage, jolted bodily off our seats, and our heads would bump against the top of the car before we dropped back again.

Our limbs got bruised as we were thrown backwards and forwards against the sides of the car or mixed with the luggage at the bottom. A tin of Huntley & Palmer's biscuits jumped clean out of the window at the back of the car and disappeared. This almost caused tears. There were rivers to ford and unstable bridges to cross. Then, too, something continually went wrong with the car itself; with a sudden jerk it would come to a halt and the chauffeur would spring from his seat and send Droog underneath to find out what was wrong. Droog would go under, come out covered with mud and give his report. After a short consultation they would both get back to their seats and we would re-start. Again there would be a jerk and a sudden stop, again they would get down, and again Droog, patient and longsuf-fering, would be pushed in a most ignominious manner under the car, come out muddier than ever and give his report; once more they would mount, but only for a short distance would we proceed before the whole business was re-enacted. The chauffeur, a good soldier and anxious to carry out his orders to get to Rashka quickly, would run round the car and ejaculate: "*Pas de chance, mon Dieu! pas de chance.*"

That night we rested at an inn at Ushtsche, a village south from Kraljevo. Four of us occupied a small room whilst the men of our par-ty slept in the car. The common rooms and passages of the inn were filled with soldiers, wrapped in their great coats or blankets, sleeping on the floor. We stepped over them to reach our room, Before we got to Ushtsche we had travelled for some time after dark, the hillsides at points being ablaze with fires. These were at the encampments of Aus-trian prisoners who were being taken away from the country. Early next morning we were astir and on the road to Rashka, which we reached in the afternoon during a heavy rainfall.

Rashka, a small town, stands at the junction of three valleys on the borders of the Old and the New Serbia. Through one end of the town, a stone's throw from the market place, runs the river which, up to the close of the Balkan war four years ago, divided it from Turkish territory. On the hillside, across the river, and seen clearly from the market place, stand the old Turkish look-out towers which command the roads from the valleys as they enter the town. In character Rashka is more of a village than a town, but it has a very spacious market square; its houses, like those in most Serbian towns, are low lying.

For a time we waited in the market place whilst Johanovitch and Milan found the chief of the police, who later placed a schoolroom at our service. The food stores we had brought were sparingly used as but little else could be bought in the place, so many people with the same wants as ourselves had already passed through. Two of us only had bedding—blankets for the others were coming in the ox waggons—this we divided as best we could and slept on the floor.

Having brought us to Rashka the chauffeur was under orders to return to Kraljevo to fetch others. The first journey had, however, exhausted the petrol and more could not be obtained. He and Milan went to Novi Bazaar as they were told they might get some there, but the journey was made in vain and the car had to remain in the market place, where it served as a bedroom for Droog.

It seemed an unkind fate which, a few days later, brought the chauffeur's chief to Rashka. This gentleman was very annoyed because the car was not in good working order and said it was due to the chauffeur's luggage. This luggage, which stood in our schoolroom, consisted of one very small plain wooden box some two feet square, which contained nothing but a dictionary, a little bundle of letters from and photographs of his family and a yard or two of ribbon in the French national colours. And this was responsible for the breakdown; it did indeed seem as if there were "*pas de chance*" for him. In the later stages of the retreat both his feet were frozen. He suffered greatly and for three months was in a hospital. He is now with his mother in his native town in France.

The site for our new camp was chosen, but it was found that the Serbs, if they made another stand, would have to make it farther on. Dr. McMillan and Sister Price, together with Dr. Milanovitch, a Serb, fitted up a dressing station where soldiers, as they came through, could get their wounds re-dressed. Similar work was done by other members of our unit on the road, and at Vitanovatz and Kraljevo as they came through.

After the first few days our school was turned into the military headquarters and we went to live in a three-roomed Turkish house near the dressing station. Madame Milanovitch often came to the dressing station where her husband was engaged and to see us in the Turkish house; we became great friends. Rashka was not their home. They, like us, were but passing through. Madam Milanovitch, a dainty little lady with beautiful dark eyes and tiny white hands, looked quite out of place in the rough and tumble of the retreat. Up to that point she had journeyed in a carriage, but now, as it was increasingly difficult to get horses or oxen, she feared it would be necessary to travel on foot when the time came to leave Rashka. In readiness for this eventuality she had a pair of her husband's boots ready for her use and had shortened one of her skirts. She shewed them to us and said that when she put them on her husband had said she looked "Quite like an Englishwoman!"

For a fortnight we stayed in Rashka, and during this time it seemed as if the whole male population of Serbia, native and foreign, passed through. One day the place would be packed with people, the next day they would be gone; again the town would be equally crowded, but with an entirely different set—so it changed from day to day. In every street, at every corner, by the river and in the market place fires were lighted. The wooden fence round the church was pulled down and burned for firewood. . At every turn animals were killed and everyone seated round these little fires seemed to be either killing, cutting up or cooking—sometimes roasting whole—a sheep, a cow or a pig. This gave a ghastly touch to the scene.

The crown prince came with his soldiers; he walked through the streets and chatted to everyone. French flying men were our neighbours and camped with their machines on the hillside quite near our house. Big encampments of Serbian soldiers came with their horses and oxen, settled for a night, or a day, and vanished only to be followed by others. Members of the Government came through and Serbian officials of all degrees, the foreign *attachés*, foreign missions; hundreds of young Serbian lads came too and each night the floors of cafes and every other available building were covered with them.

They entered the town in the evening and left at daybreak the following morning. Our own marines, with Admiral Trowbridge, were there from Belgrade. Then, too, there were thousands of Austrian prisoners. Among the latter we recognised and spoke to several who had been our orderlies at Kragujevatz; there was one who had worked with me in the same hospital ward. The Scottish Women's Unit stayed for a few days on the hillside below our house. Members of our own unit, including the Lapovo group, came too and passed on.

Every square inch of floor space in our house was covered by sleeping forms at night—all were packed in with mathematical precision. Apart from our own unit, which varied in number from day to day, we always had lodgers. Lone figures from other units were waiting every night till our people were settled, and we would then fix them up in vacant spots and share our blankets with them. When there was an extra pressure we seriously considered the possibility of tying them up in their blankets pudding fashion and hanging them on hooks to the rafters. Our meals too, as our beds, were shared. The inhabitants of the town were very friendly towards us. One day we bought some nails in the market place and the shopwoman would take no payment for them. "No," she said, when it was offered, "you are helping our soldiers."

Here news came to Milan that his brother was killed in battle against the Bulgarians. This made him very sad and he was very anxious to go to Kruchevatz for a couple of days, where his family lived, to see his mother. We were quite willing that he should go, but the military authorities would not grant him leave. The French chauffeur, a good companion in adversity, on many an occasion turned his sadness to laughter. Johanovitch (the Montenegrin) went out daily to out-lying peasants' houses to buy us food, which was increasingly difficult to obtain. The stream of people through the town at last ceased and of the inhabitants the women only remained.

Our turn at last came to go and our little group was broken up. Dorothy Brindley went off one morning just before dawn with some members of another unit *en route* to Novi Bazaar and Montenegro; Dr. McMillan and Sister Price left with Dr. Milanovitch to work in a dressing station, at the halfway stage, on the Mitrovitza Road. The chauffeur joined some of his own countrymen; and Milan departed with another section of our unit. My lot was to journey to Mitrovitza with Doctor Iles and a nurse in charge of an invalid member of our unit who had had the bad luck to be inside her bullock waggon one day when it capsized. News reached us before we left that a member of our unit, Sister Clifton, had been accidentally shot; the bullet had passed through both lungs and then through her arm. She was taken first to a hospital, then brought on a stretcher to Mitrovitza. Here she developed pneumonia and had to remain. Dr. Iles, Dr. McMillan, an orderly, and Sister Bambridge, a great friend of hers, stayed with her. All were shortly afterwards taken prisoners by the Austrians and later, when Sister Clifton was well enough to travel, sent by them to Switzerland.

Serbia, especially through Shumadia, is a beautiful country in which to "*trek*," hilly or mountainous throughout, intersected by many rivers, well wooded, and everywhere covered with a rich vegetation, which gives warmth and colour. After nightfall one saw by the roadside, on the river banks and the hillside, the blaze from hundreds and hundreds of little fires, each with its group of campers, and, just before dawn these fires would die slowly down and shadowy figures could be seen moving about, packing up their bundles ready to take to the road again at break of day.

The road to Mitrovitza runs parallel to the river. The first night we slept on hay under cover of a leaking tent at the halfway stage which we reached after dark. No sooner were we asleep than we were awakened again by heavy rain. To sit up was the only means of keeping one's head dry, and to draw up one's feet the only way to keep them out of a pond. Consequently a strictly vertical line was necessary the whole night. A gloom was cast over this little camp because in another tent a member of the Scottish Women's Hospital Unit lay dying. A day or two before, the motor car in which she was travelling ran over a precipice not many yards distant. She was brought to the camp suffering from terrible injuries to her head.

At daybreak, before leaving, we went to her tent; she was delirious and moaned with pain. We were told that she could not recover. She died two days later and was buried on the hillside just above the camp. May she rest in peace. The road from the half-way stage to Mitrovitza runs round a mountain with a deep precipice on one side; it has many sharp curves and at certain points was washed away by the heavy rains, and was so narrow that only one vehicle could pass at a time; it required the greatest skill to drive round these sharp broken curves. Many accidents occurred and we saw motors—big lorries, as well as other vehicles that had run over the side sticking at all points on the slope and lying at the bottom abandoned.

Mitrovitza is Turkish in character and quite other than Rashka. Between Kraljevo and Rashka many small differences were noticeable; the oxen were of a smaller breed and one saw men in white homespun more often than in the brown. But here in Mitrovitza the whole aspect was different. The minarets of the mosques were dotted over the town, the streets were narrower and more winding, and the secluded dwellings were surrounded by high walled gardens and courtyards. It was quite different from the Serbia we had known; for five centuries it had been under Turkish rule. The streets were literally packed with a dense crowd garbed in many varieties of colour and costume. It was a difficult task to walk even for a few yards. Oxen and people were so tightly packed together. The mud was appalling!

A hospital stood on the highest point of the town on the bank above the river, and from our tent, which the chief of the hospital had given us permission to erect in the hospital grounds, we could get a view of the town and surrounding country. It seemed impossible to find clean ground, and later we left the tents and slept in a room the Serbs put at our service in a big government granary where hundreds of bags of maize were stored. Running over the whole length of this building was a loft and here hundreds of Serbian youths were housed each night. Overhead we heard the sound of their many feet night and morning.

My duty here was to act as housekeeper and provision members of our unit as they came through. To shop was difficult. Johanovitch—the Montenegrin who had left us at Rashka to travel with his wife and daughter—we again met; he helped me and we both spent much time searching for food. The chief of the Military Hospital gave us an order for bread from the bakery, and later gave us orders too for rice, beans and meat. Sugar we bought at a shop in the market place, but could get only a small quantity at a time and that only at a certain hour of the day. Wood was scarce too and the smallest fire we made in the open space in front of the building had literally to be held from an invading army with their pots and kettles. A fire once made was never left until we had finished our cooking, but we let many strangers boil their pots and pans at the same time, every inch of space over and round the fire being thus fully utilised.

After a few days' stay and with the greater number of the unit already ahead, we—about twenty in number—with Dr. Curcin as leader, took the southern road in bullock waggons through Vuchiturn over the Kossovo Plain to Prishtina and Prizrend.

We crossed the Plain of Kossovo—that historic ground where in 1389 a great battle was fought between Serbs and Turks, and on the battlefield of which the rulers of both countries fell. The Turks were the victors, and that whole strip of territory, the Old Serbia, passed under the dominion of Turkey. This land thus wrested from Serbia and held under alien rule for five hundred years, was regained but a few short years ago after terrible sacrifice of human life. Now again it was passing from Serbia's control, and over the ground where their forefathers had fought the Serbian army was now retreating, hoping against hope for the point to be reached where they could make another stand against the invader. The soldiers did not like to leave; they said "We have been defeated before, but we have never run away." Each would have been far happier had the order come to turn back, even though it had meant certain death.

The second day out from Mitrovitza, and as we crossed this Plain, a snow blizzard burst upon us in all its fury, and an icy wind blew across our track. There was no shelter. The slow ox waggon procession moved on in what seemed a never ending journey. To the right, to the left, in front or behind, right away to the line where the sky and earth meet, nothing could be seen but a vast stretch of snow-covered land. Nothing was there to suggest food, warmth or rest; to stay was to die.

We each had an ox waggon to sleep in which also carried a portion of the stores; but after the first day, owing to breakdowns, we had to share our waggons. The blizzard took the back out of one waggon and the roof off another. Still another went over bodily into the river and was abandoned.

Everything we afterwards wanted seemed to have gone down the tide in that waggon. There was much water to cross, both rivers and flooded land. It was a pitiful sight to see the Serbian lads, many of whom were wretchedly clad and badly shod, trying to get all the warmth they could from the small woollen scarves round their necks and blowing their hands to keep warm. Being on foot, they had to wade ankle-deep, sometimes almost knee-deep, through these stretches of water, and as they came out the other side the icy wind would freeze their soaken garments to their feet and legs.

Being almost the last to come over the road we saw the wreckage of all that had gone before. It seemed a veritable road of death. Broken down vehicles of all shapes and sizes were lying everywhere. They had stuck in the mud, fallen down banks and over bridges into the rivers, with wheels off and shafts broken. A tragic sight on that awful road was the dead and dying animals. When oxen and horses could go no further, when they dropped from hunger—all animals were hungry—want of rest or broken limbs, they were unharnessed and abandoned. Everywhere, sitting, standing, lying in all positions, some already dead, and others still waiting for the kindly hand of death to touch them, the animals lay and slowly the snow covered them.

Never once throughout that long journey were we to be freed from this ghastly sight. As well might one have tried not to see the stones in the road as to have endeavoured to avoid them. Many of the dead animals were flayed. Sometimes patches of skin only were taken off. Dogs were gnawing them, and people were cutting pieces from their dead bodies. Everyone seemed to be carrying a lump of raw meat in their hands till the day's journey was over and it could be cooked on their little fire. In the midst of these horrors people slid quickly back to the primitive stages of existence. All were hungry, and other food was scarce.

One night on the road to Prishtina and Prizrend we were given a big brown tent which had been taken from the Austrians. It was riddled by bullets and let in the rain. We slept soundly and woke early the next morning to find, many of us, that our beds were in pools of water. For some reason we could not continue our journey that day, and with the prospect of a second night in the tent we lighted a large fire in the centre, dried our clothes and bedding, and turned the tent, despite the smoke from the wood fire, into a comfortable dwelling. Another shelter we got on the way was at Prishtina. Here a Turk gave us a room in his house. We were grateful as the journey that day had been a very cold one and snow was deep on the ground. Our host shewed his hospitality by bringing a charcoal brazier for us to warm our hands and sat with us round it chatting about the journey.

When the last of our party arrived the room was very full, and as uncomfortably hot as outside it had been uncomfortably cold, so two of us descended to an empty room on the ground floor which opened on to a yard. Our host said we might sleep there. To see what was on the floor or in the yard was impossible as we had but a dim light, so we slept on the window sill which was fairly wide and shivered. We had arrived quite late in the night, and started off again long before daybreak the next morning. This stage of the journey was taken very quickly, and but scant time allowed for rest for either animals or people as we were almost within range of the Bulgarian guns.

Some hundreds of prisoners from the gaols passed us at dawn during a short halt we made by the roadside for breakfast. They were tired, emaciated, hungry-looking men, and a large number of them had heavy iron chains fastened to their legs. They walked with difficulty. The reason they were chained, we were told, was because they had been rebellious or had tried to escape. As they passed, two men in the ranks called out "Good morning" in English. Eight men, spies or deserters, we were told, were shot as we entered Prishtina.

A few hours after leaving Prishtina and within a few miles distance of each other, five men were stretched out stiff and lifeless across our path. Nobody took any notice of them: all passed by, just stepping over or round the dead bodies. The driver of my ox waggon caught my glance as we passed the second man, but the only comment he made was "*Niye dobro*" (not good). One man by the roadside in an apparently dying condition was taken by Dr. May into her waggon. She wrapped him in blankets and gave him food and took him on to Prizrend, where she handed him over, on the high road to recovery, to the care of a Serbian hospital.

One saw, too, many hungry Austrians; these men were taken away in batches of hundreds at a time, and there were always individuals who could not keep up with the others. They were permitted to drop out and make their way down to the coast as best they could. Many

127

of them were literally starving. They would come to us with clasped hands begging for bread, but we had nothing to give them. It was terrible, for in many cases we knew that within the next few days they would be dead, and would never see their homes or their country again.

All this misery and all the many roadside tragedies were happening not because anybody was going deliberately out of their way to be unkind to anybody else, but it was the inevitable result of war and invasion. And so long as countries recognise war as a legitimate means of settling their differences, so long as countries are greedy for their neighbours' territory, these tragedies will be re-enacted.

From Prishtina to Prizrend it is a long climb, the road looping itself many times before the summit is reached. At the top a magnificent panorama of mountains, the Crnoljeva, lay open before us; our road then for a long distance dropped steadily before reaching the town. Prizrend is Turkish in character and more eastern even than Mitrovitza. The streets are narrower and more winding; they are paved, as are all the streets in Serbian towns, with large, round, uneven cobble stones, but intersected by many water channels which are to be seen oftener in the towns of Old Serbia. There seemed scarcely space to enter the town; the streets, packed more densely than those of Mitrovitza with a cosmopolitan crowd, were almost impassable. Our drivers, oxen and waggons camped outside the town with soldiers and many other refugees. We were able to secure rooms in a Turkish house and stayed for two nights. The street crowds were fascinating. Several of us climbed to the castle and found there a big crowd of Austrian prisoners. Many of the buildings were stored with guns and ammunition; everything suggested war.

Here news came that the road through Monastir was menaced by the Bulgarians and any hope of getting through to Salonika was futile. To double back on our track was the only thing to do; not on the same road, but on the one leading to Ipek. Had we known when at Mitrovitza that the Bulgarians would cut off the road at Prizrend we might have gone to Ipek by a much shorter route. The Austrians, too, were advancing rapidly; it was doubtful whether they or we would reach Ipek first.

The first day back from Prizrend was one of the pleasantest and most peaceful of the whole journey. There was a warm gentle breeze, the sun shone, and stretching away into the distance on either side of the roads were fields and grassy slopes. Peace seemed to have come again to earth, and for a while there were fewer people. A long procession of Serbian artillery was about an hour's distance ahead, and behind were other ox waggons and a miscellaneous crowd of refugees. One of the earlier and sad sights on this road were groups of tired, worn and crippled horses and oxen.

Djakovitza was our objective on leaving Prizrend, and it was a far longer journey than we had expected. As night fell the oxen grew tired and hungry, and progress was slow; several of the last waggons which contained eight of our party got cut off from the others. Two of the oxen broke down and as the waggon had to be left behind we spent some time in transferring the most urgent portion of its contents to the other accommodating waggons. The oxen were brought on at their own pace by their driver. After pressing forward till about eight o'clock all hope of catching up with the front section of the party that night vanished, and a halt by the roadside was made. There was not much hay in the waggons, but all that they contained the oxen ate, and two big fires were made for the drivers and ourselves.

Later the moon came out and lighted up the countryside. Our group of eight sat round the fire, drank tea and told stories. Some Serbs came across the fields to our fire with their "*guyde*" and played native music; whilst they played our Serbian orderlies placed their hands on each others shoulders and thus in a row kept time with the music in a rhythmic swaying dance. An Irish nurse sang some sad Irish songs. Then the fires died down and we turned into our ox waggons for sleep; the drivers lay on the ground near the shafts with their heads almost touching those of their oxen.

At two o'clock the journey was resumed and we travelled on through the night. The soft light of the moon gave everything a touch of unreality. Nothing besides our five waggons with their occupants was on the road. About an hour later the ancient bridge that divides Serbia and Montenegro was crossed, and a little further on the road bent sharply over a second bridge. Two of us who had walked ahead waited here for the others, and felt all the beauty and all the strangeness and silence of this moonlit world steal over us—it was as though we were standing in Eternity.

Djakovitza was reached the next morning, where the first section of the party were already established in a room adjoining a mosque. Here a two days' halt was made and our stores and equipment further reduced. At Prizrend much had been given to the hospitals. Several oxen were exchanged for ponies, as they would be wanted later for the mountain journey.

The shops, especially those in the older part of the town across the river, were full of interest. They were workshops and retail shops combined. Copper and tin goods of all kinds, jewellery, white skull caps, and a variety of other articles were being made in full view of the customer: there was also some beautiful embroidery. In every shop two or three men were either at work or sitting round a charcoal brazier. One or more charcoal braziers seemed to be part of the equipment of each shop; also three-legged stools, which were like halves of six-legged stools, and some practice in sitting on them was necessary before a sure balance could be maintained. Two of us bought three-penny knives—not because we wanted them, but because we wanted to sit on a three-legged stool, warm our hands at a charcoal brazier and converse with the proprietor.

The call for prayer came from a neighbouring mosque. Many men came and all took off their shoes in an outer lobby before they entered the inner chamber. From this lobby we saw the back view of a kneeling row of worshippers, who at intervals bent forward till their foreheads touched the floor. No women came. Mosques have no seats, but the floors are carpeted. The streets were full of children and both boys and girls looked very quaint in their wide printed cotton trousers. They were as full of run, energy and mischief as other groups of town children in any part of the world. The men, especially those who were elderly, presented quite an elegant appearance in their white home-spun suits, trimmed with black braid. The trousers were fitted in closely to both leg and ankle, and then made to spread gaiter fashion over the foot; this, together with their white stockings and black slippers, gave their feet a flat appearance. The dress was very handsome and the wearers were refined in manner and appearance.

On the open spaces near the town were large encampments of Serbian soldiers. A fair amount of food could be bought and there was an air of comfort everywhere. It seemed to us then as if Montenegro had been wrongly described as a barren foodless country. An extraordinary number of graveyards are to be seen in and near Djakovitza—there are acres of grass-covered mounds.

Between Djakovitza and Ipek another blizzard swept over the land and the ground was white with snow. A night was spent at the monastery at Detchani. Serbia has many of these monasteries with their spacious yards, which can give shelter to numbers of men, animals and vehicles at the same time. All are surrounded by high walls and can only be entered through the big heavy gates.

Before the monastery was reached the oxen had grown very tired, and again two waggons were cut off; they were fated to get behind breakdowns the whole day. One waggon contained hospital equipment and the other Sister Price and myself. Towards nightfall the road, snow-covered and intersected by many streams, that could not be seen until they were reached, became very difficult. Darkness fell, the oxen moved slowly, and the drivers, always patient, plodded steadily on by their side; hunger and tiredness made no outward difference to them, they were as capable of endurance as were the oxen they drove.

Throughout the day we—Sister Price and myself—had walked, but when the darkness fell the driver urged us to get inside the waggon as the road was narrow and uneven and the waterways dangerous. To catch up the others we felt was impossible, and so settled ourselves for the night. Later we were wakened from a sound sleep by Doushan's voice (one of the Serbian orderlies) telling us we were at the monastery. Although we were hungry and cold, and warmth and supper were inside the monastery, we felt that in being disturbed we had a real grievance. A large room hung with portraits of the founders of the monastery and Slav saints was placed at the disposal of our party, of whom the majority were already in bed.

Eight of our party left early the next morning to finish the journey alone. It was necessary for them to reach England quickly and so it was arranged that they should go first to Ipek, take the few ponies assured to us there, and not suffer unnecessary delay through lack of transport for the others. They took leave of us at the monastery just after dawn. Thick snow covered the ground. On the second morning the rest of us left, and experienced the coldest journey of the trek.

People on the road were in agony—so cold, piercing and merciless was the wind. It blew across the ice bound roads, till they were polished and sparkling as glass. Animals slipped and fell at every turn, many broke their limbs and were left by the roadside. A peasant woman was on the road with two children—one she carried and the other ran by her side crying with the cold. A Serbian officer took them all in his conveyance and put his coat round the children. Fortunately the distance to Ipek was not great and long before dusk the journey was ended.

A room in the house of a Montenegrin was placed at our disposal by the authorities. Had we known its history we might not have entered with quite the same spring in our steps. A few hours after our arrival a man came in and did not seem at all inclined to go away. He seemed anxious to know when we would leave and we thought him very fussy, and although he was quite at home in the house we looked upon him as a fellow refugee. Then we found we were mistaken and that he was the owner of the house. He had come straight from prison, where he had spent some time for the murder of his wife, to find his house lent to us. He was quite polite, but eager for our departure. The crime was committed, we learned, in the very room we occupied.

Ipek might have been the North Pole, so thickly encrusted was it in ice. The slaughter of oxen was terrible and far ghastlier even than in Rashka. Their work was done, they were not wanted on the mountains—for the road ended here—so people were lavish in the slaughter, and at every few paces warm steaming blood ran across the streets. Pack ponies were scarce and the demand for them great—everybody wanted them for the mountain tracks. It was necessary to stay in Ipek till such time as they could be bought or secured in exchange for oxen. All the ponies were weak, lean and hungry; they had been worked to their utmost and not given sufficient food for some weeks.

The number eventually secured was quite inadequate. One pony between two people was the order. On asking what weight a pony could carry, we were told about one hundred and thirty kilograms. As, however, we could not guess the weight by just looking at the amount of stuff, an assortment of the most necessary articles was made. A ground sheet and blankets for two people and two people's share of food (all the food was divided and each made responsible for their individual share), the driver's blankets and the pony's corn, enough to last for a certain stage of the journey, had to be taken; also various pots and pans. When all these oddments were collected and my pony was loaded, the cargo made an impressive appearance.

A Serbian boy, who had not even half a pony, hung his blanket and boots on the saddle. Instead of kit for two, the pony was thus to carry the kit for four, to say nothing of his own corn. He therefore began the journey by sitting down, and it was probably the wisest course he could have taken. He was at once "undressed" and got on his feet. The weight was reduced and more expertly packed, and with a more cheerful expression the pony then lined up with the others and kept his head up well to the journey's end.

It was in Ipek that we again met Mrs. Stobart and the other members of the unit who had been with her. They came into the town with a section of the army and camped by the roadside between us and the monastery. Two of us called to see her and stayed to eat. In spite of the cold the camp was snug, the motor cars were drawn round to make an enclosure, and in the centre of this was the fire. Tarpaulins were hung round to break the wind. Later we called at the monastery to see several others who were leaving her there to link up with us.

From Ipek there are two routes—one *via* Rosji, longer than the other but a better road; on the shorter road the tracks were bad and dangerous. Dr. Curcin brought us over the latter route, as the other, though a better road, would be more crowded and chances of food and accommodation less. The short route, however, turned out to be equally long, for owing to the heavy snowfall and cold winds the tracks were icebound and the way beset with difficulties.

The main travellers on this route were Serbian soldiers who were leading their horses. One horse had a large copper boiler strapped to its back, and this boiler dogged our steps from Ipek onwards. During the first stage of the mountain journey, before the track narrowed, we saw motor lorries lying at the bottom of steep precipices. They were sent over purposely so they should not fall into enemy hands; many cars, waggons and guns were destroyed.

The last night at Ipek came the news that the Austrian army had been repulsed at Mitrovitza and that the Serbs would follow up the advantage thus gained by a big offensive movement. It was said that instead of continuing the retreat it might be necessary the next morning for all to go back to Mitrovitza. The effect was electrical, each pulse quickened and the light of renewed life shone from every face. We slept that night not knowing what the morning would bring. When morning came, and with it the order to go forward, everyone fell into the old pace and that new light vanished.

The mountain tracks were very bad for the ponies, especially where the water dripped from overhanging rocks and made large holes in the snow. The drivers sounded the depth of these with a stick; although they were sometimes not very deep the unevenness of the bottom would often cause the ponies to slip. Points, too, were dangerous where an ascending path curved inwards, for after passing the curve at its inmost point a pony would often lose its foothold and slip backwards, the driver keeping hold of the bridle would be pulled off his feet, and as the two slid backward towards the edge of the track a cry would be raised and the other drivers would leave their horses and come to the rescue; this help, though always in time, never seemed to arrive till the twelfth hour when we had had our fill of horror in witnessing these hairbreadth escapes.

Nikola, a Montenegrin whom we had engaged at Ipek, acted as our advance agent across the mountains. He would start earlier than we to find a suitable camping place for the night, always allowing for us to reach it by nightfall. Once, however, he did not rightly gauge the distance, and we had a short journey after darkness had fallen. The path was narrow, steep, slippery and frozen hard again after its slight thaw in the midday sun. A nurse in front of me lost her footing and slipped forward into the darkness; in trying to save her my foothold was lost and a horse behind me slipped also. The three of us, none the worse for our adventure, landed at the bottom of the slope in a heap. There was laughter at our expense, as on the downward journey we had addressed the horse in Serbian and asked him to "*Chekka molim*" (stop, please), when it was as impossible for him as for us to stop.

Exact information as to distance could never be obtained. Terms of measurement were not in miles or kilometres, but in hours or days. Then, too, whilst in Montenegro it was always necessary to distinguish between a Serbian and Montenegrin hour or day. The Serbs walk well, but the Montenegrins—whose country is one vast mountain—take enormous strides and cover the ground very quickly. Equally tall as the Serbians, the Montenegrins are perhaps of somewhat slighter build, their legs are free from the skirt of an overcoat, and they do not appear to wear so many clothes. Sometimes we could get a room in a Montenegrin peasant's house, and the members of the family would always be intensely interested in our movements and would sit in our room the whole time whilst we were going to bed or rising in the morning, there was no privacy.

The majority of us, however, always preferred to sleep round our camp fires under the stars. We bathed in the streams, and washed our clothes, too, in the same manner when time permitted. The summit of the first mountain range, the Tchakor, was passed at the close of the second day. At any point of this mountain journey (which took us nine days) when looking backwards or forwards soldiers in single file could be seen on the looped tracks; they made a thin moving and never-ending line on the vast slopes of those mighty mountain sides.

Andrejevitza was reached about the fifth day. Many thousands of soldiers had already gone through. On the top floor of a cafe, which was built against a hillside, we succeeded in getting a room where, when asleep, we resembled little mounds in a closely-packed grave-yard. A wretched night was spent; in the violent wind we expected the hinges of the casement to snap; and on the landing outside our door an imbecile Turk wandered about the whole night.

Early morning saw us again on the road. Our journey this day was one of only two or three hours, for we found a farmhouse on a beautiful hillside, where a halt was made till the next morning. It was a glorious day, warm sunshine and no wind. In a stream that rushed down the hillside we bathed and washed our garments, which we hung on the hedges to dry. There was plenty of wood for our campfires. We slept in the open air, and felt clean once more.

Another delightful stopping place was the last stage before coming to Podgoritza; this too was a farm. The house was very old and consisted of but two rooms, a wide flight of steps, quite palatial, led to the entrances, two doors side by side (and looking like one) led into the separate rooms. In one room the family lived and the other was used as a storeroom. In the latter, amongst much else, were dried vegetables and fruits, corn and hay, bins of hide, horn and string. Numerous families of rats and mice were there too as discovered by several of our members who slept in the room. A river ran within a few minutes' walk from the house and here again we were able to bathe, and wondered if the folks at home would shiver if they knew we were bathing in the open air in December.

Much fishing is done by the Montenegrins, but a rifle instead of a net or line is used. One man will wade in the river and with a long pole prod and poke in the banks and under the stones; another will walk along the riverside some distance up the bank with a rifle and shoot the fishes as they swim away after dislodgment. Some fishermen came one day when six of us were bathing and fired their rifles within a few yards of where we were; it was slightly disturbing as we felt there might be some inaccuracy in their aim, but we soon discovered that they knew what they were about; they shot their fishes and passed on as if we were not present. Snowdrops grow wild on the Montenegrin mountains between small thickets so that they cannot easily be gathered. Our common garden sage grows too on the mountain sides.

In Podgoritza it rained heavily. The Hotel des Balkans gave us shelter and meat meals; bread we had to supply or go without. We were very hungry, not that we were ever quite without food, but it was impossible to get the right kind. Maize bread and meat were our stock foods. The bread was full of sand which got between our teeth and was not only very unpleasant but caused dysentery amongst many of our members. If at any time other bread could be obtained, it was given to those who suffered these ill effects. A deep craving for fruit and sugar was experienced by all, but these were only very rarely obtainable. Rice and raisins, it was rumoured, could be got in Podgoritza; for half a day, however, we searched the little town from end to end, visited each shop and looked in all the bins and boxes, but without success. A tantalising but amusing incident happened in the Podgoritza market.

A peasant woman had some "*kymak*" (soft cheese) to sell at eight *dinars* (*francs*) per kilogramme. We were quite prepared to pay this sum, but as she was about to serve us a police official interfered and said the price was exorbitant and that she must not sell for more than half the price. Then she would not sell at all, and we who wanted the "*kymak*" had to be content to see her close the basket and fold her arms across the top. At intervals during the day we pressed her to sell. Even bribery was tried and we offered the eight *dinars* when the official was not looking, but to no avail; she was adamant. Later the official said she could sell for five *dinars*, but then she raised her price to nine *dinars* and we were still baulked of attainment. A similar instance occurred when we wanted potatoes from another seller.

An official in answering inquiries about the despatch of letters said, "Oh yes, you can write your letters and can post them, but the boxes are never cleared." A sporting instinct at once prompted us to write to our friends. In Serbia all letters were franked for us by the government; not being sure whether this would hold good in Montenegro, we took no risks but bought stamps and handed our cards over the post office counter. This was on December 13th, and they reached London quite safely five weeks later. The last letter received from London at Kragujevatz was dated October 3rd. At Mitrovitza a copy of the *Westminster Gazette* for October 15th was seen. In this was a paragraph to the effect that in view of the possible invasion of Serbia arrangements had been made for the transference of the seat of government to Mitrovitza. Not only had the transference taken place, but the government had long since gone again.

King Nikola I. of Montenegro passed through the streets of Podgoritza; he rode a tall, light grey horse and wore a large light grey cloak which reached to the stirrups. His gold decorations and orders and the polished silver stirrups shone from their background of grey. A body-guard of soldiers on foot encircling the horse and rider were also resplendent, but in a slightly lesser degree. The sun, after the heavy rain, came out brightly and as the little group crossed the bridge they glittered and sparkled in its light. For a moment it seemed to lift them above the common muddy condition of the streets and people, and no one might have been surprised to see a halo suddenly appear round the king's head like a saint in days of old. They passed and we continued our walk across the bridge in the mud, with our vision still a little dazzled. Several of us attended a short intercession service here at a Catholic Church, the building was very small and the floor was of bare earth. Opposite the Hotel des Balkans and across the little boulevard was a public garden with flowers and trees, the first attempt of the decoration or laying out of a town that we had seen for a long time.

The evening before we left Podgoritza we held a "reception" at the Turkish Schools, across the river from our hotel, where the drivers and ponies were sheltered. A big wood fire was made in the school yard and some cabbage we had bought was put into two empty kerosene tins and turned into soup. Two of us went across early to prepare the meal and the others who were the guests followed later. They came through heavy rain and almost ankle-deep mud and we met them at the school door, shook hands and said "How do you do?" and "so good of you to come." The soup in the meantime was served straight from the kerosene tins to the guests as they came up in turn.

When leaving Kragujevatz we had each brought, as instructed, a knife and fork, spoon and a plate and cup. These had long since disappeared and the receptacles now presented by the guests for soup were of strange and various shapes. All of us returned later through the mud and rain to the hotel. Our orders were to be ready and sitting on our baggage by six o'clock the following morning, and six o'clock found us carrying out the instructions to the letter. The conveyances came two hours later, and after a good deal of doubt had arisen as to whether they would appear.

The road now lay over flat country to the Lake of Scutari, and waggons were again used. These were like shallowly scooped out lorries with no covering. The bundles of blankets and kettles were tossed in, and we sat on the top of these with our feet hanging over the sides. Rain fell and the wind was cold. The horses, two to each waggon, were the strongest we had seen during the whole journey and resembled the rather small, sturdy, thick-set type of Russian horses, wearing the wide harness set with brass so often seen in pictures.

Instead of going to the head of the lake, we made for a point a little way down on its eastern side. The boat that we expected did not arrive, and after waiting for some hours we took refuge in a big, empty

137

granary, where we stayed till noon of the next day. In the centre of the wide stone floor we lighted a fire. Here we took in lodgers—members of another unit who could not find shelter. We "entertained angels unawares," for later our lodgers drew from their possessions a small tin of Demerara sugar when they found we had none, and gave us each a spoonful for our tea those of us who had already had our tea—took the sugar in our hands and used our tongues as spoons.

The next day the sun shone brightly as we sat on the little quay waiting for the boat to arrive, and the wind had dropped. High overhead for a long time a Taube circled and hovered like a huge silver bird against the sky. Loud explosive reports could be heard startlingly near, and we were told that Scutari and San Giovanni di Medua were being bombed. This we found later was true.

Twelve British marines were waiting too for the boat. They were the last men down from Belgrade, who had been left to cover the guns. They were hungry, weak and tired, and one of them fainted from sheer exhaustion and had to be lifted on board the boat. They said they had been firing by day and trekking by night. Food was discussed, and one man said that raw cabbage was "fine tackle." The long beards which they had grown, and which they disliked exceedingly, gave them a strange appearance. We were all glad to meet each other, and the cockney accent of one man who hailed from the "New Cut" was as music to our ears. Later on board, as they sat round the cook's stove watching some water boil, they leaned against each other's shoulders and sang "Who killed Cock Robin?"

The lake journey took about seven hours. Failure to get a boat would have meant a further five days' journey by the side of the lake. Many people told us that this road was beset with danger, as the Albanians would at any point sweep down the mountain side and slaughter us for loot, that they were bandits and would wipe us out and that nothing would ever be heard of us again. Later we learned that other members of our unit had gone over the road and nothing had happened beyond the terrible hardships caused by the bad condition of the road and fording of many rivers.

When on the lake some curious person suddenly asked "What day is it?" It sounds as if to answer would be easy, but all knowledge of days and dates was lost. No newspapers, letters or business appointments came our way, and one day seemed very much like another. On asking such a question the answer one would get would be "They say it's Wednesday," or "They say it's Sunday." Our diarists got the nearest, but did not help us much, as they were always so hopelessly in arrears and had to go back such a long way before they could get a basis for their reckoning. So when this question was asked on the boat some one turned to a Serbian officer to see if he knew, and he turned to a captain who was asleep, shook him with "*Kapitan, Kapitan,*" and asked him: *Kapitan* was about to answer when he had his doubts, rubbed his forehead and passed the question on to somebody else. Thus the question went round and no one, either Serb or Britisher, could give an answer.

Gipsies, also refugees, were on the boat, and someone suggested they should be asked to play a violin one of them carried. When approached on the matter the Serbian officer, who was an old man and very sad at leaving his country, said, "No, with my permission no one shall play music, the time is too sad." Soon afterwards, when our marines sang "Cock Robin," although they sang quietly to themselves, we felt that the colonel would not perhaps understand. So it was explained to him that it was not light-heartedness but sadness that made the marines sing. It was the way of British people to sing sometimes when very depressed; it disguised their feelings to others and enabled them to present a bold front to the enemy. He smiled, and we hope he understood.

Scutari was reached after nightfall and we walked into the town from the landing stage. Several two-wheeled ox waggons—quite different from any we had previously seen—took our blankets and kettles and other belongings. These were placed in the waggons so badly by the Albanian drivers that they were shaken out, and two of our members who walked behind the procession came up with their arms full of miscellaneous oddments that they had picked up from the road. The night was spent in a school, where hot soup was given us, and three rooms with a plentiful supply of hay put at our disposal. After breakfast the next morning we went by invitation to the British Consul's house. Tea, in real china cups, and tobacco were handed round. We sipped the tea and rolled cigarettes as we waited the consul's arrival.

Two-wheeled ox waggons, like those of the previous evening, at which the Serbs laughed and said they had seen nothing like them before—came to take us to San Giovanni di Medua. The oxen were a much smaller breed than those used in Serbia and they kept their noses almost to the level of the ground as they pulled the waggons. The drivers, who were Albanians, carried long sticks but never struck the oxen; they conducted them by pointing this way or that. The oxen seemed to understand their driver's every word and movement. In these drivers an entirely new type of human being was presented to us, and two days only in their company was not sufficient time for us to grasp "their point of view," and so the meaning of many strange happenings remained unrevealed.

To begin, it was extremely difficult to make them understand that we wanted to ride in the waggons, although we could not imagine for what else they thought we had hired them, and quite half a day vanished before a start could be made. Our instructions, on leaving the consul's house, were to walk behind the waggons to the point where the drivers got hay. The first waggons contained our blankets, and with these many of our Serbian escort walked; the second contained hay for the oxen; and in the third set we tried to ride. But for some unexplained reason the Albanians wanted to fill all the waggons with hay and desired that we should walk.

The Albanian language is quite other than Serbian, so that neither we nor the Serbs were capable of pressing our point of view. The Albanian sergeant who was in command of the drivers could understand a little Serbian and at times conversed with one of our men. But they seemed to keep in the background during these very trying negotiations.

Finally, imagining that deeds might speak louder than words, we took the law into our own hands and commenced to climb into the waggons and to the top of the truss of hay that filled them. Objection was taken to this and, when nearly at the top, my driver took hold of my foot and pulled me down again into the road; the others were treated in similar fashion. After repeated efforts we at last got in and the journey was resumed. All went well until the drivers suddenly seemed to discover that we were not seated on the right spot, and motioned us with angry glances to move this way or that way. Sometimes it was very difficult to know which way they wanted us to go. Two expressions only seem possible on the faces of the Albanian drivers—one a broad smile, the other a tragic scowl; there is nothing between the two and they never get from one to the other, but the expression is the one or the other.

When two of us were seated comfortably on the top of the hay in our waggon suddenly the driver's face took on the tragic scowl; he came to the side of the waggon gesticulating wildly. It was clear that he wanted us to move, but it was not at all clear as to where he wanted us to go. First we moved to the front of the waggon, which was quite wrong and he was very angry, then to the back, but this was wrong too and he was angrier still, then, not knowing what else to do, we sat down on the very spot we had left. His expression was radiant. The drivers too treated us as if we were inanimate. When sitting or lying peacefully in our waggons the driver's coat or a piece of wood would suddenly land on us. The driver would see a nice dry piece of wood by the roadside, pick it up for his camp fire in the evening, and toss it into the waggon without troubling to see where it would fall—if it fell on us, well, that was our look-out.

That night, through the delay in the early part of the day, we found it impossible to reach the point where we had intended to camp. Progress was extremely slow, as the land was heavily flooded, and instead of roads there were vast tracks of watery waste to cross; the mud was inches deep. Dead horses were everywhere, many in an advanced state of decomposition, and the odour at points was almost unbearable. The night was spent at an Albanian farm. Our host gave us a room, in which he lighted a big fire. He showed us great kindness, and refused to take any money in return for the hospitality he gave. A very early start was made the next morning to make up for the time lost. Again we had some difficulty in getting into the waggons. There was a slight improvement in the roads, and many of us walked. The drivers walked the whole way through the mud and water with bare feet. At one point where a halt was made to feed the oxen, there were patches of dry grass-covered ground. Here the drivers washed their feet in the pools, took off their top pair of trousers and hung them on the waggons to dry.

One of the surprises an Albanian driver gives is the number of pairs of trousers he wears. It does not seem to matter how many pairs he takes off, there is always a pair underneath. Yet the Albanian does not appear to be over-weighted with clothes; he is of slight build, alert, nimble, and has all the lithe agility of a panther. His garments are made of a cream homespun—the under garments of a thinner texture than the outer ones, and his head is swathed in handkerchiefs.

San Giovanni di Medua was reached on the night of the second day out from Scutari. We were told that an American sailing vessel—though we might have to wait some time for it to come—would take us across the Adriatic. On our arrival we found that an Italian vessel which had run unexpectedly into the harbour, having discharged its cargo of food, was about to leave again. The captain was in a great hurry to be off, but hearing of us he sent a message that although he already had on board one hundred and twenty members of different units, including some of our own who had taken the road before us, who had waited at the port five days for a boat, he would take us if we were quick.

We were hurried from our ox waggons into rowing boats without having time to say goodbye to the little group of Serbian soldiers who had tramped that long journey with us from Kragujevatz. Masts of sunken food ships dotted the harbour, and we rowed between them to the Italian steamer in the bay. The vessel moved off before those of us in the last two boats were able to get on board. We shouted, but to no effect, and realising we must wait for the next ship turned to row back to the shore.

Suddenly we were hailed, and the vessel stopped—someone had probably prevailed on the captain to wait for us; we rowed up quickly and were hauled on board with all the despatch and unceremonious-ness of bits of luggage. The boat was crowded but we sat down on the deck and slept through the night, with the waves breaking over us from time to time. By eleven o'clock the next morning, after a twelve hours' passage, the Adriatic was crossed and Brindisi lay before us set in glorious sunshine. Italian, British and French battle craft of all kinds lay in the Brindisi waters and, massed together as they were, made an impressive show of strength and power. Every vessel appeared to have had a washing day, for each had lines stretched across its deck hung with rows of very homely useful garments.

It was all rather like a dream to step ashore. After the rough and tumble of camp life and the long journey made under such primitive conditions along rough roads, across snow covered plains, and over wild mountain ranges untouched by the hand of man, it was now as though one had stepped on to the stage of a theatre or into a child's toy picture book. Nothing seemed real—the real world was the land of mountains and hunger we had left.

Italian officials wearing handsome uniforms and immaculate linen, and rings on their elegant white hands, came across the quay to meet us. We were hungry, tired and unwashed, with the dust and mud of a seven weeks' journey on our boots, and our clothing a patchwork of each other's garments. When the officials saw us they went back and cleared all the women and children off the quay. It was as though they had said "This is not a sight for members of the weaker sex, this is man's work to disembark these wild women." The Italians were very kind and placed first-class travelling accommodation at our disposal.

Through Italy and across France we journeyed, and then from Havre to Southampton for home. Before the British Government would permit us to land at Southampton we had each to fill in a paper containing many questions; one of these was "Give exact reason for coming to England."

We were back again with home, friends and comforts before us, yet it was a sad home coming, and gladly would we have retraced our steps. Our thoughts went ever back to the Serbian soldiers whom we had left on that inhospitable Albanian coast. The men who had come down the long road from Kragujevatz and who had borne privation and danger without flinching, men who were hungry, tired and worn, without proper clothes or other equipment, and whose boots were almost off their feet. Throughout the long journey every step brought us nearer to our homes, but took them ever farther from theirs. Our hearts and our thoughts went out to them and we longed for the time when they would be back again in their own country; back once more in those little homes that we knew so well, dotted throughout the length and breadth of Serbia, reunited to their women folk and their children, able to enjoy, as never before, all the blessings, all the comforts and all the joys that life can yield. We longed too for the time when all the ghastly business of war will be over and done with for ever, and sanity come to the peoples of the earth.

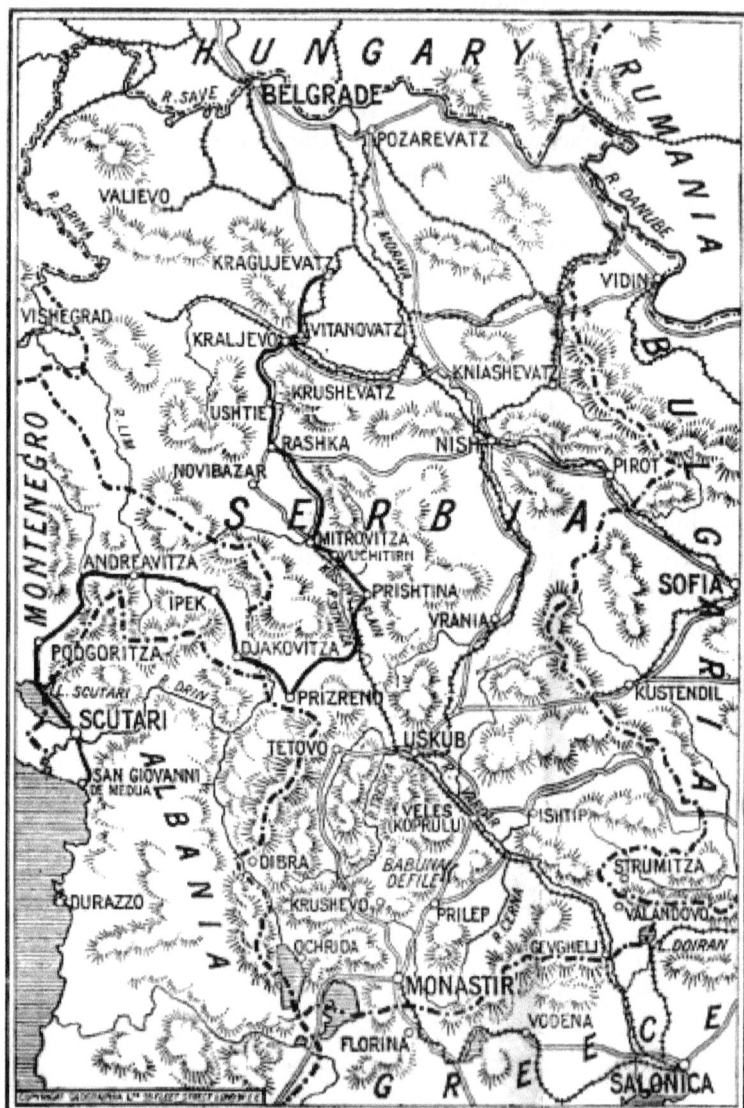

ROUTE OF RETREAT: SHOWN BY THE BLACK LINE

Note on Serbian History

Of the pre-Balkan history of the Serbs but little is on record except that they are of Slav origin and lived as an agricultural people in the Carpathians. Owing, however, to unrest caused by invasion of their lands by the Goths in the seventh century, groups of these virile tribesmen came down into the Balkan Peninsula, where they rapidly spread and intermixed with the Latin and Greek peoples. The early part of their Balkan history was largely influenced by Byzantine culture, and under its influence Christianity supplanted their old Pagan faith.

For their greater strength and common protection the tribes came together as a people and made repeated efforts, eventually successful at Rashka in the ninth century, to found a Serbian State. From that time onward, but with many ups and downs and much internecine strife, they pressed steadily forward developing their territory and power, and in the fourteenth century were the strongest people in the Balkan Peninsula and could be reckoned as one of the important powers of Europe.

At that time, however, the Turks were making determined efforts to penetrate further into Europe, and encouraged by their earlier successes in the southern part of the land—where on the Maritza in 1371 King Vukasin and 60,000 Serbian soldiers were slain, and also to anticipate an allied move against them by Serbia, Bulgaria (a province of Serbia at that time), and the State of Bosnia—made a big sweep forward and challenged the Serbs to a battle (1389) on the Plain of Kossovo. With no lack of courage, although the forces were three to one against them, the Serbs boldly answered the challenge and fought so valiantly that despite the tremendous odds they faced history might have had a different tale to tell had not a traitor in their camp left the field with his men when the battle was in progress.

The battle is chronicled as a religious one between Christianity and the Islamic faith. The rulers of both lands, Knez Lazar and Sultan Amourath I., were killed, and of the Serbian soldiers but few were left. All the land except Montenegro passed to the Turks, and under their sway Serbia was gradually robbed of her freedom. Then for over four centuries Serbia as a nation disappeared from the map. The people were in a state of vassalage, and their lands and rights as individuals were taken from them unless they conformed to the Islamic faith. The brightest boys were taken to Constantinople and trained in the *"Janisseries"* to fight for the Turks. Yet, spite of much suffering the Serbs kept the spirit of their independence alive and never forgot throughout those long years that they had once been a nation. Their history, told in unwritten ballads, was passed on from one generation to another. The great deeds of their people were thus kept alive in their memories, and the children, born in vassalage, learned that they belonged to a great people who were once free.

Successful rebellion against Turkish authority began in 1804 when the independence of Belgrade was won. This was lost again in 1813. but regained two years later. Thus steadily, bit by bit the grip of the alien ruler was loosened. Eventually in 1913, at the close of the Balkan War, the Serbs having regained the lands of old Serbia and Macedonia freed themselves entirely from the Turkish yoke and stood again as a nation before the world, looking to the time when the 7,000,000 of their people who were living under Austrian rule (Austria annexed Bosnia from Turkey in 1908) would win their freedom and all would unite under a common government.

Austria objected to Serbia's freedom; it was to her interests that Serbia should remain small and helpless. She not only objected to the possibility of giving up the provinces in her possession but she wanted Serbia too, or at least a highway through it with an outlet in the Ægean Sea, and was violently opposed to Serbia having a port anywhere. Serbia's good fortunes had thus to be checked at the outset and so another war was forced upon her. So, scarcely had Serbia freed herself from her Turkish foes before she found herself confronted by Austria and involved in another struggle.

Independence so dearly purchased from the Turks was thus lost again, and in the last months of 1915 Serbia passed into Austrian hands. Not that Austria was stronger than the Turk or could accomplish what the Turk could not, for alone she could not have successfully invaded Serbia. Three times she tried and three times she failed; but it was only because Germany and Bulgaria came to her aid that this fourth attempt succeeded.

Again as on Kossovo Plain Serbia has fought with three to one against her, but this time it has been three countries. Again she has been overpowered and her men and boys between the ages of fifty and fifteen are in exile; and the women of the country, strong, capable and courageous, are facing the enemy alone, and are representing the Serbian nation within their country today. The end is not yet, but those who know the men and women of Serbia know that there is in their character a virile element of independence and individuality that long centuries of foreign rule could not obliterate and that their land today is only invaded, not conquered. Austria and Germany both want Serbia the former for reasons already stated; the latter to link up the Austro-German Empire with Constantinople and the East. Serbia wants her own land and people under her own control for the quiet, orderly development of her race.

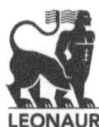

ALSO FROM LEONAUR
AVAILABLE IN SOFTCOVER OR HARDCOVER WITH DUST JACKET

THE WOMAN IN BATTLE *by Loreta Janeta Velazquez*—Soldier, Spy and Secret Service Agent for the Confederacy During the American Civil War.

BOOTS AND SADDLES *by Elizabeth B. Custer*—The experiences of General Custer's Wife on the Western Plains.

FANNIE BEERS' CIVIL WAR *by Fannie A. Beers*—A Confederate Lady's Experiences of Nursing During the Campaigns & Battles of the American Civil War.

LADY SALE'S AFGHANISTAN *by Florentia Sale*—An Indomitable Victorian Lady's Account of the Retreat from Kabul During the First Afghan War.

THE TWO WARS OF MRS DUBERLY *by Frances Isabella Duberly*—An Intrepid Victorian Lady's Experience of the Crimea and Indian Mutiny.

THE REBELLIOUS DUCHESS *by Paul F. S. Dermoncourt*—The Adventures of the Duchess of Berri and Her Attempt to Overthrow French Monarchy.

LADIES OF WATERLOO *by Charlotte A. Eaton, Magdalene de Lancey & Juana Smith*—The Experiences of Three Women During the Campaign of 1815: Waterloo Days by Charlotte A. Eaton, A Week at Waterloo by Magdalene de Lancey & Juana's Story by Juana Smith.

NURSE AND SPY IN THE UNION ARMY *by Sarah Emma Evelyn Edmonds*—During the American Civil War

WIFE NO. 19 *by Ann Eliza Young*—The Life & Ordeals of a Mormon Woman During the 19th Century

DIARY OF A NURSE IN SOUTH AFRICA *by Alice Bron*—With the Dutch-Belgian Red Cross During the Boer War

MARIE ANTOINETTE AND THE DOWNFALL OF ROYALTY *by Imbert de Saint-Amand*—The Queen of France and the French Revolution

THE MEMSAHIB & THE MUTINY *by R. M. Coopland*—An English lady's ordeals in Gwalior and Agra duringthe Indian Mutiny 1857

MY CAPTIVITY AMONG THE SIOUX INDIANS *by Fanny Kelly*—The ordeal of a pioneer woman crossing the Western Plains in 1864

WITH MAXIMILIAN IN MEXICO *by Sara Yorke Stevenson*—A Lady's experience of the French Adventure

AVAILABLE ONLINE AT **www.leonaur.com**
AND FROM ALL GOOD BOOK STORES

07/09

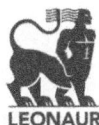

LEONAUR

ALSO FROM LEONAUR
AVAILABLE IN SOFTCOVER OR HARDCOVER WITH DUST JACKET

A DIARY FROM DIXIE *by Mary Boykin Chesnut*—A Lady's Account of the Confederacy During the American Civil War

FOLLOWING THE DRUM *by Teresa Griffin Vielé*—A U. S. Infantry Officer's Wife on the Texas frontier in the Early 1850's

FOLLOWING THE GUIDON *by Elizabeth B. Custer*—The Experiences of General Custer's Wife with the U. S. 7th Cavalry.

LADIES OF LUCKNOW *by G. Harris & Adelaide Case*—The Experiences of Two British Women During the Indian Mutiny 1857. A Lady's Diary of the Siege of Lucknow by G. Harris, Day by Day at Lucknow by Adelaide Case

MARIE-LOUISE AND THE INVASION OF 1814 *by Imbert de Saint-Amand*— The Empress and the Fall of the First Empire

SAPPER DOROTHY *by Dorothy Lawrence*—The only English Woman Soldier in the Royal Engineers 51st Division, 79th Tunnelling Co. during the First World War

ARMY LETTERS FROM AN OFFICER'S WIFE 1871-1888 *by Frances M. A. Roe*—Experiences On the Western Frontier With the United States Army

NAPOLEON'S LETTERS TO JOSEPHINE *by Henry Foljambe Hall*—Correspondence of War, Politics, Family and Love 1796-1814

MEMOIRS OF SARAH DUCHESS OF MARLBOROUGH, AND OF THE COURT OF QUEEN ANNE VOLUME 1 by A. T. Thomson

MEMOIRS OF SARAH DUCHESS OF MARLBOROUGH, AND OF THE COURT OF QUEEN ANNE VOLUME 2 by A. T. Thomson

MARY PORTER GAMEWELL AND THE SIEGE OF PEKING *by A. H. Tuttle*—An American Lady's Experiences of the Boxer Uprising, China 1900

VANISHING ARIZONA *by Martha Summerhayes*—A young wife of an officer of the U.S. 8th Infantry in Apacheria during the 1870's

THE RIFLEMAN'S WIFE *by Mrs. Fitz Maurice*—*The Experiences of an Officer's Wife and Chronicles of the Old 95th During the Napoleonic Wars*

THE OATMAN GIRLS *by Royal B. Stratton*—The Capture & Captivity of Two Young American Women in the 1850's by the Apache Indians

AVAILABLE ONLINE AT **www.leonaur.com**
AND FROM ALL GOOD BOOK STORES

07/09

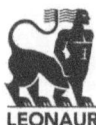

ALSO FROM LEONAUR
AVAILABLE IN SOFTCOVER OR HARDCOVER WITH DUST JACKET

DOING OUR 'BIT' *by Ian Hay*—Two Classic Accounts of the Men of Kitchener's 'New Army' During the Great War including *The First 100,000 & All In It.*

AN EYE IN THE STORM by *Arthur Ruhl*—An American War Correspondent's Experiences of the First World War from the Western Front to Gallipoli and Beyond.

STAND & FALL by *Joe Cassells*—A Soldier's Recollections of the 'Contemptible Little Army' and the Retreat from Mons to the Marne, 1914.

RIFLEMAN MACGILL'S WAR by *Patrick MacGill*—A Soldier of the London Irish During the Great War in Europe including *The Amateur Army, The Red Horizon & The Great Push.*

WITH THE GUNS *by C. A. Rose & Hugh Dalton*—Two First Hand Accounts of British Gunners at War in Europe During World War 1- Three Years in France with the Guns and With the British Guns in Italy.

EAGLES OVER THE TRENCHES by *James R. McConnell & William B. Perry*—Two First Hand Accounts of the American Escadrille at War in the Air During World War 1-Flying For France: With the American Escadrille at Verdun and Our Pilots in the Air.

THE BUSH WAR DOCTOR by *Robert V. Dolbey*—The Experiences of a British Army Doctor During the East African Campaign of the First World War.

THE 9TH—THE KING'S (LIVERPOOL REGIMENT) IN THE GREAT WAR 1914 - 1918 by *Enos H. G. Roberts*—Like many large cities, Liverpool raised a number of battalions in the Great War. Notable among them were the Pals, the Liverpool Irish and Scottish, but this book concerns the wartime history of the 9th Battalion – The Kings.

THE GAMBARDIER by *Mark Severn*—The experiences of a battery of Heavy artillery on the Western Front during the First World War.

FROM MESSINES TO THIRD YPRES by *Thomas Floyd*—A personal account of the First World War on the Western front by a 2/5th Lancashire Fusilier.

THE IRISH GUARDS IN THE GREAT WAR - VOLUME 1 by *Rudyard Kipling*— Edited and Compiled from Their Diaries and Papers Volume 1 The First Battalion.

THE IRISH GUARDS IN THE GREAT WAR - VOLUME 2 by *Rudyard Kipling*— Edited and Compiled from Their Diaries and Papers Volume 2 The Second Battalion.

AVAILABLE ONLINE AT www.leonaur.com
AND FROM ALL GOOD BOOK STORES
07/09

www.ingramcontent.com/pod-product-compliance
Lightning Source LLC
Chambersburg PA
CBHW021005090426
42738CB00007B/661